More praise for

SOMETHING FOR THE PAIN

"The searing honesty of *Something for the Pain* makes the heart glad and breaks it at the same time. Austin's clarity is sobering; his humanity is simply staggering. This chronicle is the unsentimental account of a man who has seen men and women at their worst—and at their best. He has been to the Valley of the Shadow of Death but refused to stay there. Reading Dr. Paul Austin's riveting story makes me proud to be a human being."

—Randall Kenan, author of *The Fire This Time*

"*Something for the Pain* is remarkable for its compassion, humanity, and scrupulous honesty."

—Michael Collier, author of *Dark Wild Realm*

"It turns out there are all kinds of things about working in an ER that most of us haven't learned from TV or having sat in one. In *Something for the Pain*, Paul Austin—the ER doc you'd hope to get if something really bad happened—tells us, vividly and with uncommon candor, how, if you aren't careful, saving people's lives can make you sick."

—Ted Conover, author of *Newjack*

"Courageously peeling away the layers of his life—both professional and personal—Austin tests and finds his limits as a doctor and a father. And when he does, he shows us something universal about how we all break and heal each other and ourselves."

—Rachel DeWoskin, author of *Foreign Babes in Beijing*

"*Something for the Pain* has everything you want in a medical memoir: urgencies, emergencies, life-or-death. And, yes it 'goes behind the scenes'—so shockingly, at times, that it borders on confession. But the real revelations here are more subtle; Austin, writer as much as physician, can turn the simplest procedure into an occasion for elegy, paean, or profound meditation, phrased with the elegance of a Thoreau. Blood, yes, and pain aplenty—this is a book about the body. But it is also about the spirit, about trauma in all its definitions, about what it costs to heal and be a healer, what it truly means to save a life."

—David Bradley, author of *The Chaneysville Incident*

"An intensely personal and truthful account of life as an emergency physician. Great reading for all who work in an acute care environment. If you are considering a career in emergency medicine, you must read this book."

—Eugenia Quackenbush, MD, FACP, Assistant Professor of Emergency Medicine, UNC School of Medicine

"Austin gives a stunning account of the chaos of the emergency room, the constant drama of urgent situations calling for immediate and decisive action. He pulls us inside the chronic exhaustion ER docs fight against and fully engages us in the difficult juggling doctors do."

—*Boston Sunday Globe*

"Buy this book! I simply could not put the book down. These are not Hollywood rewritten vignettes. . . . This is real-life emergency medicine. . . . Buy it, read it, share it, and enjoy!"

—*Academic Emergency Medicine*

SOMETHING FOR THE PAIN

SOMETHING FOR THE PAIN

COMPASSION AND BURNOUT IN THE ER

PAUL AUSTIN

W. W. Norton & Company
New York London

Printed in the United States of America
First published as a Norton paperback 2009

For information about special discounts for bulk purchases,
please contact W. W. Norton Special Sales at
specialsales@wwnorton.com or 800-233-4830

Manufacturing by Courier Westford
Book design by Rhea Braunstein
Production manager: Anna Oler

The Library of Congress has cataloged the hardcover edition as follows:

Austin, Paul, 1955–
Something for the pain : one doctor's account
of life and death in the ER / Paul Austin.
p. ; cm.
ISBN 978-0-393-06560-2 (hardcover)
1. Austin, Paul, 1955– 2. Emergency physicians—United
States—Biography. I. Title.
[DNLM: 1. Austin, Paul, 1955– 2. Emergency Medicine—Personal
Narratives. 3. Emergency Treatment—psychology—Personal Narratives.
4. Physician-Patient Relations—Personal Narratives. 5. Physicians—
Personal Narratives. WZ 100 A937a 2008]
R154.A92A3 2008
616.02'5092—dc22
[B]

2008020114

ISBN 978-0-393-33779-2 pbk.

W. W. Norton & Company, Inc.
500 Fifth Avenue, New York, N.Y. 10110
www.wwnorton.com

W. W. Norton & Company Ltd.
Castle House, 75/76 Wells Street, London W1T 3QT

1 2 3 4 5 6 7 8 9 0

TO SALLY

CONTENTS

Introduction: Tool Bag 9

PART ONE

Night Shift 15
Still Hurting 24
The Caring Curve 35
Something So Personal 43
Declaring a Patient 59
Ventilator 72
Among Savages 83
Face-to-Face 101

PART TWO

Mrs. Kelly 113
Splinters 137
Tucker Put His Gun to His Head 143

Longing for Sleep 155
Seeking Rehab 165

PART THREE

Somebody's Baby 185
Sleeping at My Mother-in-Law's 196
Sleeping Quarters 210
Gunshot Wound to the Chest 222
Why Don't You *Do* Something? 234
Something for the Pain 261
The Devil Is a Beautiful Man 274
Rotating Shifts 282

Epilogue 291

Acknowledgments 295

INTRODUCTION: TOOL BAG

I CARRY a black canvas tool bag to work. I copied the idea from David,* one of the other docs in our group. My bag is filled with the essential things that help me make it through a shift—a bag lunch, a snack, and a can of V-8 Juice—it can get so busy there's no time to go to the hospital cafeteria, but I can usually sneak down the hall to the break room for five minutes to wolf down a sandwich. My bag also has a Littman stethoscope. A reflex hammer with an orange rubber head shaped like a triangular tomahawk. A PalmPilot loaded with a drug database, and some other programs I don't use much. A *Harriet Lane Pediatric Handbook* and a *Sanford Guide to Antimicrobials*—we have a bookshelf in the doctors' dictation booth, but the books seem to wander off, and it's frustrating to need a piece of essential information and not have it. Especially in an emergency.

I have a copy of the new CDC guidelines for treatment of sexually transmitted diseases—they've recently discovered that gonorrhea is resistant to Ciprofloxacin. I also have a bottle of

*All the names and identifying characteristics of patients, staff, and friends have been changed to protect their privacy.

Hemmocult developer because I sometimes can't find it in the cabinet over the sink in the nurses' station; a roll of silk tape; and a pair of trauma scissors.

I still have the Welch Allyn otoscope/ophthalmoscope kit I bought in medical school twenty-two years ago, but its zippered case fell apart during residency. I made a replacement out of walnut. It looks like a cross between a jewelry box and a miniature carpenter's toolbox. I made a snug little compartment for the handle, and a special place for the ophthalmoscope head. There are five circular holders for the graduated plastic earpieces. I made a tray for the stainless steel ear curettes—fine, long little spoons—that are so handy for getting wax out of ears and beads out of noses. In the lid of the box, I keep a laminated diagram of the ear canal, the tympanic membrane, and the middle ear. I always show it to the child's mother before I start scooping with the curette, so she won't worry that I'll poke a hole in the eardrum. Under the otoscope handle, I keep a pair of delicate alligator forceps—precisely machined of brushed stainless steel. The jaws have tiny little teeth, which are perfect for grabbing a moth's wing or a cockroach's leg after the insect has crawled down into someone's ear.

I keep a bunch of refills for my ballpoint pen. A portable telephone I clip to my scrub pants. A leather change purse I got in Honduras. A bottle of generic ibuprofen. Laminated copies of the NIH Stroke Scale and the Mini-Mental Status exam.

I also keep a spiral-bound copy of the research papers I had to read for the most recent annual recertification exam. I highlighted the articles that I may need in a hurry: the treatment of acute ischemic stroke, the use of dexamethasone in adults with meningitis, the treatment of pediatric head trauma, and community-acquired pneumonia in children. I also keep a checkbook in my turn-out bag in case the nurses are collecting money for someone's birthday or baby shower, or if a coworker we like is leaving, and we want to buy them a cake to put in the break room on their last day.

Every day when I get to work, I put my lunch in the dorm-sized refrigerator in the docs' office, and grab three teabags from my locker. I put a granola bar and a Ziploc baggie of grapes or cherry tomatoes next to one of the computer terminals in the nurses' station, and then drape my stethoscope around my neck, put a few of the business cards that I give each patient into the pocket of my scrub top, the PalmPilot into my back pocket. Then I tuck the reflex hammer into the waistband of my scrub pants.

Finally, I take a blank three-by-five index card and across the top write the date, and the day of the week. I work rotating shifts, which are assigned without regard to weekends, so it can be difficult to remember if it's Tuesday or Wednesday. On the card I will make a list of the patients I'm taking care of. I slip the card into the pocket of my scrub top, grab a chart, and go see my first patient of the shift.

PART ONE

NIGHT SHIFT

During the day, it's not so bad. But at night, sleepy mistakes make it difficult to keep people moving safely and quickly through the emergency room: a tired lab technician misplaces a tube of blood, a nurse flushes a urine sample, or I flip through page after page of test results on a patient with a productive cough and shortness of breath, unable to remember if I have looked at his chest X-ray.

I picked up Emma Lowery's chart from the rack under the clock in the nurses' station, and clamped my mouth against a yawn. I clicked my pen and noted the time: 2:57 A.M. I walked toward her room. A homeless man with matted hair snored on a stretcher in the hallway, and in the next cubicle a patient from a nursing home filled the department with the stench of liquid stool oozing from the edges of his adult diaper. A phone rang unanswered.

At this time of the morning—two, three, four o'clock—lonely people seek solace in the fluorescent light of the emergency room. If you've been to a twenty-four-hour grocery store late at night, you may have seen the same people. They hesitate, put a can of soup back on the shelf, then take it down again and put it back in the cart. Refugees from the daylight world, they move with the timidity of those whose lives don't mesh with others'.

Night is the time when the lucky people get to sleep. But toothaches throb more in the dark, and backaches become unbearable. People in pain abandon their restless beds and flee their empty kitchens. They go out into the night, in search of comfort.

"Good morning," I said to the young woman as I entered her cubicle. "I'm Paul Austin, one of the ER doctors. How can I help you?" I pulled the curtain closed behind me, and sat in the chair next to her stretcher.

She sat with her legs crossed, and her hands in her lap. Her auburn hair was pillow-flattened and her face was that of a child woken too soon from an afternoon nap. As she talked, she motioned vaguely with her hands, hammered silver bracelets jingling up and down her forearm. "I've been having this headache for a month now," she said, rubbing her right temple with her fingertips. "I've been to the ER once and my own doctor twice. He sent me to an ear, nose, and throat doctor. He said that it wasn't my sinuses. No one can help me." She ran her fingers through her hair. "I'm so spacey and confused. It's just not like me."

I nodded, and listened as carefully as I could. So far, the ER had been busy, but not out of control. I'd been running several charts behind all night, but was beginning to catch up. The shift, which had begun at 9:30 P.M., was my third of three nights. The other ER doc had gotten off duty at one o'clock, and I was by myself until seven in the morning, when I would lurch gratefully back into the daylight. I've been an attending physician in the ER for ten years, and nights are still scary: one bad wreck involving multiple patients can put a strain on the entire department. No one works as efficiently at night as they do during the day.

The *Exxon Valdez* oil spill, the Three-Mile Island meltdown, and the chemical plant explosion in Bhopal, India, all happened on the night shift. I just wanted to make it to daylight without hurting someone.

As soon as she said she'd had the headache for a month, my interest began to wane. *If it took a month to get this bad, it'll probably be okay for at least a few more hours. Why did she wait until two o'clock in the morning to come in?* I have an abiding fear that while I'm grinding through an ER full of non-emergencies, there's someone I've not gotten to whose coronary arteries are clotting shut, or whose inflamed appendix is about to burst.

I began the physical examination, but was called away to another room for a patient with chest pain. Then the paramedics wheeled in two patients from a motor vehicle accident. I tried to get back to the woman with the headache, but sicker people kept coming in.

At six o'clock, Lisa, one of the nurses, said, "Paul, you need to make a decision about that girl in room eight."

"Yeah, I know," I said. "There's nothing wrong with her." I thought about discharging her right then, but I hadn't done much of a neurologic exam, and hadn't examined her retinas. I yawned. "Lemme go take another look at her, and then we'll let her go." I knew her exam would be normal, but it would only take a couple of seconds.

I went back to Ms. Lowery's cubicle. "I need to look in the back of your eyes. There's an important part of your retina, and I can't stop looking until I see it clearly." I took the ophthalmoscope from the bracket on the wall as I talked. "I know the light's bright, but the stiller you hold your eye, the quicker I'll be done. Okay?"

She shrugged. "Sure." She fixed her blue eyes on the far wall, and waited.

I tilted my head back, so I could peer through my bifocals and the ophthalmoscope, and saw the red reflex, like a flash-bulb eye on a color snapshot. I moved in closer, until my cheek almost touched hers. I could smell her sleepy breath. Peering through her pupil like a keyhole, I turned the dial, *click, click, click*, until her retina came into sharp focus. Tracing the retinal arteries and veins back to where the optic nerve attaches, I expected to see a pale white disc against a deep red background. The junction between white and red is normally well defined, crisp. In the back of Ms. Lowery's eye, streaks of white blurred into the red of the retina. *Damn*.

"Now the other eye."

She pulled her hair back again. "Am I holding my eye still enough?"

"Yeah, you're doing great." The ophthalmoscope is so bright it's uncomfortable for the patient, and some people sigh loudly as I peer into their eyes, or pull their head away just when I'm about to see the disc. I appreciated her cooperation.

I peered through the ophthalmoscope into her other eye. We both held our breath, while I clicked the retina into focus. The disc margins were indistinct in that eye, too.

Blurred discs are a sign of increased intracranial pressure. It could be a brain tumor. Or it could be something much less serious.

I leaned back, and put the ophthalmoscope back in its holder. "Ms. Lowery, the back of your eye is called the retina, and in the middle of the retina is the optic disc, where the optic nerve connects. Yours are swollen. I need to get a CAT scan of your brain."

She frowned. "Is it bad?"

"It could be something simple, or it could be something serious. Let's get the CAT scan and see." I didn't want to make it any more scary than it already was.

Rick Earnhardt, my relief, showed up at 6:59 A.M. He's the quintessential ER doc—smart, funny, and decisive. "How was your night?" He took a sip of coffee from a Styrofoam cup.

"Not as bad as it could've been. I was just getting ready to discharge the woman in room eight—came in about two o'clock with a headache that she's had for a month. I thought it was bullshit until I went back and looked at her retinas."

"And?"

"Her discs are blurred."

"Oops." Earnhardt hunched his shoulders and pulled his head to the side. "Dodged that bullet." He grinned. "You want me to follow up on the CT?"

"I've got some charting to do." I glanced at my watch—7:03. She should get back from CT by 7:20, and I'd get the results by 7:45, so I could probably get out of the ER by 8:00. I'd been hustling all night, hoping to get out on time. I was tempted to let Earnhardt deal with it, but I felt bad for misjudging her. "I'll stay."

Thirty minutes later, the CT technician wheeled Ms. Lowery back to her cubicle, and then walked over to the nursing station. The technician sat down next to me, and pulled her chair close. "She's got a mass this big," she whispered, forming a circle with her thumb and middle finger. "It's the size of a golf ball. The radiologist's going to call you in a minute with the formal report, but the mass is pretty obvious."

The radiologist called. I spoke with Dr. Davis, the neurosurgeon on call. He asked a few questions, and said he'd be right in. I was glad I'd be turning Ms. Lowery's care over to him. Some of the on-call doctors try to dodge admissions. They look for reasons that I should send the patient home or to another hospital—anything to keep from having to come in and deal with the admission. But Dr. Davis seemed ready to take care of whatever problem I called him about. His approach made my job easier and inspired confidence he'd take good care of Ms. Lowery once he got to the hospital.

I sat in the dictation booth, not looking forward to telling Ms. Lowery she had a brain tumor. But the sooner I talked with her, the sooner I could go home. I took a deep breath, and went to her cubicle. "How are you doing?" I paused at the curtain.

She shrugged and slowly scratched behind her right ear. "Sleepy. Still have the headache."

I pulled a chair a little closer to her stretcher, and sat. "Ms. Lowery, is anyone here with you?"

"No."

"Is there anyone I can call for you?" It would be easier for both of us if she had someone with her.

She shook her head again. "Not really. Why?" She squinted. "Did the CAT scan show something bad?"

"It showed a mass in your brain." I paused, to let it sink in. "I've already spoken with a neurosurgeon, Dr. Davis. He's smart, and he's nice."

Ms. Lowery nodded slowly. "How bad is it?"

"I'm not sure," I said. "Some are easier to treat than others. Dr. Davis can explain it to you better than I can. Be sure to ask him about anything you don't understand. He'll take good care of you."

Ms. Lowery slowly nodded, looking more sleepy than scared. Was she in denial, or was she relieved to finally have an answer, even if it was a scary one?

I waited. "Any other questions?" I hoped she didn't have any, because I felt sleepy and stupid.

"Not right now."

I'd done my job, but I felt bad leaving her by herself. On the other hand, if I sat much longer, I'd probably doze off. I stood and opened the curtain to leave. "Open or closed?" I asked her.

"Closed is fine."

I pulled her curtain behind me and went to the locker room, hung my stethoscope in the locker, stripped off my scrubs, and tossed them in a hamper. Wearing jeans and a T-shirt, I walked outside into the cool morning air. Dr. Davis was just pulling into the parking lot. I walked over to his car. "Good morning," I said, as he got out of his BMW.

"Good morning to you." He smiled. "Bad night last night?"

"Not as bad as it could've been." I glanced back at the hospital. "If you think about it, tell me how Ms. Lowery does." I walked to my truck, glad to be outside under a dawning sky.

When I got home, I pulled into the driveway and set the emergency brake. I sat for a moment, feeling the morning sun on my closed eyelids. I wanted to step out of my truck and into a daylight world where I didn't feel sluggish and dull, where my movements were free of the jittery imprecision of too much coffee. But I'd crossed the border between night and day too many times to expect such a quick transition. It always takes a couple of days to settle back into a normal circadian cycle.

After a string of night shifts, I lose a day just catching up on sleep. There's an empty spot on my work schedule so that it counts as a day off, but it feels more like a day of recuperation. But I can't complain; sleep lag is one of the costs of working rotating shifts, the price I pay to avoid carrying a beeper—the price of keeping home and work separate.

I walked to the house, unlocked the front door, and quietly slipped inside. I didn't smell coffee or hear movement. Everyone was still in bed, sleeping late on a Saturday morning. Part of me was relieved. I would have enjoyed a warm welcome, but I'd been interacting with people all night, and it felt good to be left alone. I made a cup of French roast decaf and poured a bowl of Cheerios.

Sitting at the kitchen table, I thought about Ms. Lowery. I was glad I'd gone back to examine her retinas. Sometimes it's skill that keeps you from making a mistake, sometimes it's luck. But usually it's just doing the drill. I hoped Dr. Davis could resect her brain mass without scrambling her personality and dulling her intellect.

I wondered how she'd face the next few days. I sipped my coffee. Would she jumble her words after the surgery? Walk with a limp? I ate a spoonful of cereal. I was glad those would be Dr. Davis's concerns, not mine.

My real concern was how close I'd come to sending Ms. Lowery back out into the night. I could imagine her standing under the lights of the ER parking lot, brushing a stray curl of hair from her face and wondering why she felt so spacey and why her headache wouldn't go away. The near miss made me wonder what other errors I *had* made. Most of the cases had been pretty straightforward and I'd been careful all night, but working a night shift is as impairing as a serving of alcohol.

I yawned, feeling too tired and dull to think anymore. Mistakes are inevitable. I'd made them in the past and would make them in the future. But I was pretty sure I hadn't this shift. And I could accept that as good enough.

I stared at the front page of the newspaper and finished my cereal, but my mind wouldn't focus. I felt my thoughts slowing, my head bobbing. I started awake, then carried my dishes to the sink. Upstairs, I took a hot shower and felt the water beat down on my shoulders and the steam rise up to my face.

Clean and relaxed, I slipped into bed next to Sally.

She murmured and shifted around to face me. "How was your night?" She drowsily opened her eyes and smiled.

"Sad." I hadn't really felt it until that moment. I shifted closer to her. "Can we be spoons?"

"Sure." She turned back over and burrowed her bottom into my lap.

The pillow cradled my head gently, my hips and shoulders eased into the mattress. I felt the weight of my body fade. The morning sun was pale through white lace curtains and the sheets were soft with Sally's sleep.

Sally turned her head to face me. "Good night," she whispered. Her breath had the same sleepy smell as Ms. Lowery's.

STILL HURTING

I'm not one of those people who always wanted to be a doctor. I hadn't even considered the possibility until I took a biology class at the University of North Carolina at Chapel Hill. I sat next to an affable guy who liked to chat as he pulled his spiral notebook from his backpack and arranged three ballpoint pens on his desk, just so. As soon as the professor began talking, my classmate hunched forward in his chair, clamped his lower lip between his teeth, and scribbled at a furious rate, trying to capture every word. He was premed.

I was twenty-seven years old, and had recently returned to college after dropping out for nine years. Although I had enjoyed the freedom of doing exactly as I pleased, I had begun to feel that my life had no direction or purpose. That's why I'd gone back to school.

The next time I saw my classmate, I mentioned that I'd been thinking about medical school. He snorted and shook his head, and held up a finger as he listed each hurdle between me and medical school. You had to have a stellar transcript. You had to do volunteer work—preferably in a hospital. You needed experience in a research lab. You had to ace the Med-Cat exam. He chuckled. You don't just *apply* to medical school. I felt my face flush as I nodded along, listening to the reasons I would never get in.

A couple of days later I met with a premed adviser to find out if it was really that hard. Turned out, my classmate hadn't exaggerated much. After the meeting I sat on the steps outside, thinking. I knew I was weak in science—before I dropped out of college I'd been an English major. My present classmates seemed younger, smarter, and better prepared, but I was pretty confident that I could outwork them.

The cold stone steps became increasingly uncomfortable. I stood and stretched. Trying to get into medical school would give me a challenge and a goal that would organize my life. I slung my book sack over my shoulder and walked down the steps. I could load up on physics, chemistry, and physiology without telling anyone I was premed. That way, I wouldn't seem foolish or arrogant, and if I didn't get in, I wouldn't have to explain it to anyone.

I ran out of money quicker than I'd thought I would, so I got a job as a nursing assistant in the emergency room of a North Carolina hospital. One Saturday afternoon, the paramedics rolled their narrow gurney toward a curtained cubicle in the emergency room. I put down the bedpans I'd been restocking, and followed them. "Gunshot wound, back of the leg," the paramedic gave his report to Julia, one of the ER nurses. One trouser leg of the mechanic's coveralls had been slit all the way up to the belt, to expose the injury. "Blew a piece of the femur out through the front." A shard of bone jutted out through the skin of the man's thigh like a curved, primitive knife. The wound splayed open, its edges as sharp as if a razor had made the incision. The muscle glistened red. The man's bare leg was skinny and pale and lay motionless against the dark fabric of his work pants. His jockey shorts were a grayish-yellow.

The man's eyes darted over to Julia. "It hurts." The corners of his mouth pulled downward. His face had a short stubble of dark whiskers; his hair was cropped close. He breathed deliberately and regularly: in through the nose and out through pursed lips.

"Grab the bottom sheet," Julia told me, "like this." She leaned forward, the stethoscope draped around her neck swinging away from her chest. Most of the nurses wore scrub pants and tops, but Julia always wore a blue scrub dress, white stockings, and white shoes.

I was new in the ER, and eager to help. I watched her closely.

Julia gathered the sheet in her hands, working more of it into her fists until they were right up against the man's body.

Two paramedics on the other side did the same. They all waited for me to get a grip.

Julia counted to three, and we whisked him over from the paramedics' stretcher to ours.

The guy shut his eyes tight and made a squeaky noise as he clutched his leg above the sliver of bone jutting out into the air. He opened his eyes and looked at me. I backed away. My throat and stomach tightened.

Julia touched the man's shoulder. "Be right back."

I hurried after her. Her brisk competence was intimidating, but she seemed willing to teach a new guy like me, and I wanted her approval. I admired the way she'd remained calm and pleasant all morning as the rescue squads brought us patient after patient, until stretchers lined our hallways. She was experienced, and could do the little extras. As she walked past a demented nursing home patient whose gown had been left awry, exposing her plastic diapers, Julia tugged it down over the lady's knees without slowing her pace, without even seeming to notice she'd done it. And in real emergencies, she knew exactly what to do.

In the closet where we stored IV supplies, she jabbed a plastic spike into the bottom of a bag of normal saline. "Here," she said. "Bring this to me when the fluid's dripped all the way through the line." She handed me the clear IV tubing. "Flush out all the air pockets." She started back to the man with the bone sticking out from his thigh, then stopped and looked back at me. "You understand we don't want to inject air into his veins, right?"

"No air," I said. "Got it."

The fluid slowly slid through the loops of the clear IV tubing. If I squeezed the bag, it would run faster. But Julia hadn't told me to, and I didn't want to screw something up. I was taking an Introduction to Physics class and could've quoted the pertinent laws of fluid dynamics, but I was afraid to squeeze a plastic bag of IV fluids. Probably better to wait the extra few minutes than run the risk of ruining the IV setup and having to start all over. I told myself to relax and enjoy the short break from the chaos in the ER. I was doing what I'd been told, and as soon as the air bubbles were out, I'd take it to Julia.

I worked every weekend in the ER and was in class Monday through Friday. The job made up for what scholarships and loans didn't pay, and gave me the chance to meet people who could write letters of recommendation for me. I was still nervous around doctors because I'd never known any, other than the pediatrician my mom took me to when I was a child. His waiting room smelled like alcohol, and had a small merry-go-round with four wooden horses, their carnival paint chipped and scarred. It didn't spin.

Every time I got a shot, my doctor handed me a stick of Juicy Fruit gum for the ride home.

The fluid in the IV line continued its slow progress. I knew the guy was hurting and needed the IV, but I couldn't take it to Julia until the fluid had flowed all the way to the end of the tubing. Finally, the last air pocket sputtered out. I ran my thumb down the little white plastic wheel that turned the IV off and hustled it over to Julia.

The guy was making louder squeaky noises in his throat—a tight sound that was more than a whimper, less than a scream.

"Big stick," Julia warned the man in a bored monotone, as she slipped the catheter into a vein at the crease of his elbow. She moved calmly as if his arm were one of the rubber models for practicing IV skills. "Gimme that," she said, holding out her hand.

I held out the bag of fluid, still staring at the end of the bone sticking out of the man's leg. It looked like a feather carved from ivory and then polished perfectly smooth, the edge tapering to an impossible thinness.

"I need the *end* of the tubing." She kept her thumb buried in the crease of his arm, pressing down on the vein to keep blood from running out onto the floor.

"Oh, yeah." I felt stupid as I snatched at the dangling end of the tangled IV tubing. "Here." I knew my rushing was making me clumsy, but I hadn't seen enough medical emergencies to be able to work efficiently.

"You'll need to untangle it," Julia told me. She looked up at the man's face. "We'll get you some pain medicine in just a minute, sir," she said. She took a deep breath and quietly let it out. "As soon as we get your IV running." She looked down at the floor.

"Thanks," he said.

I felt my face flush as I fumbled with the IV tubing. Finally it was straight, and I handed it to her.

"Thank you," she said, as she twisted the IV tubing onto the needle. She taped the plastic needle to the guy's arm, in a deliberate way, first one tab of tape, then the other. "I'll be right back with one of the doctors," she told him.

I stood beside the stretcher. *I should be doing something more to help.*

Julia came back with Kyle, one of the interns, strolling behind her in green scrubs and deck shoes without socks. Kyle had a deep tan and sun-bleached hair.

He stood at the end of the stretcher and folded his arms.

"Damn," he said, with a subtle note of amusement in his voice. He looked over at me, raised his pale eyebrows, and grinned. He stared at the bone, shaking his head. "Does he have a pulse?" he asked, all business now. He leaned over and gently placed two fingers on the top of the man's foot. I knew that, just like at the wrist, you can feel a pulse on the top of the foot, as well as on the inner part of the ankle. "Dorsalis pedis is intact." He pulled a pen out of his coat pocket and made a small "X" on the top of the guy's foot. "Lucky." He felt to the side of the ankle. "Posterior tibial's good, too." He marked that spot with his pen as well. He straightened and looked across the man to Julia. "What's his name?"

"Randal," the man answered. "Randal Meyers."

"Randy," Kyle said, "you're a lucky man."

Lucky? I looked from the bone to Kyle's face.

He frowned at the man and pointed at his foot. "I didn't really expect to find any pulses."

"I need—something—for the pain," the man stammered, between quick little breaths, "'cause it's getting—bad."

Kyle shrugged with one shoulder, and turned to Julia. "You can give him some morphine."

She left to get the medicine.

Kyle reached out his hand and brushed the side of the man's foot. "Sir," he said loudly, "can you feel this?"

"Yes," the man said.

Kyle brushed the other side of his foot. "What about this?"

"Yes, yes, yes. Am I going to get something for the pain?"

"Just a minute." Kyle's voice had an edge of irritation. "You could've trashed your nerves. I need to check them."

"I've got the morphine right here, sir," Julia said, as she returned and slipped the needle of a syringe into a port on the IV tubing. She eased in the plunger.

As the medicine began to take effect, the man relaxed his grip on his leg. He grunted, a subtle sound of gratitude and relief, then took a deep breath and slowly let it out.

I took a deep breath, too. I'd been a full-time firefighter for five years, after dropping out of college the first go-round, so I'd gotten used to emergencies, but not medical ones. We went on a few medical calls, but mostly we put out house fires. Early on, an old-timer had told me, "When you get to the fire, don't look at it. Concentrate on what you're supposed to be doing." Good advice. A fire that's burning out of control can be enthralling, and you find yourself staring at the flames dancing from the windows and bursting through the roof. It's scary and awesome. There's beauty in fire, even as it burns someone's home down to the foundation.

As a firefighter, I learned to focus my attention on the task immediately in front of me. But I'd never seen a man with a sliver of bone slicing its way up out of his leg, and the distraction—coupled with my worrying about the man's pain—had made me clumsy at the only thing I'd been asked to do to help him. If I was going to become a doctor, I'd have to learn how to deal with this kind of stuff.

"That was just five milligrams." Julia looked from Mr. Meyers's face to Kyle's.

"Okay," he said. "Repeat it if he needs it. But don't snow him." Kyle looked around the ER. "Anyone here who can sign an op permit?" He pointed to the leg. "They'll have to take this to the OR."

"Yeah, I know, but he just got here." Julia glanced toward the entrance to the ER. "Someone'll probably show up soon."

"Wait a minute." Kyle said. "He'll need to sign an op permit before he gets any morphine."

"He's already gotten it." Julia pulled the needle from the port in the IV line. "But don't worry, someone'll sign for him." She looked up at the man's face. "Mr. Meyers, is anyone coming to wait with you?"

"My brother," he said, as he eased his shoulders down until they rested on the stretcher. "My brother should be here soon." Mr. Meyers lifted his head off the pillow and looked down at his leg. "How bad is it?"

"Pretty bad," Kyle said. "But you're neurovascularly intact." He pointed to the leg. "Your arteries and nerves seem okay." He grinned. "Like I said, you're really lucky."

"Can I have something else for the pain?" His voice was less strained.

"Don't give him any more." Kyle frowned at Julia. "At least till I talk with ortho. They'll need to talk to him before we snow him too far."

"Are you okay?" Julia asked.

"I'm still hurting." He slowly lowered his head to the pillow and closed his eyes. "But not quite as bad."

"Would it feel better," I asked, "with a pillow under it?"

"No!" The man held up one hand, fingers spread wide. "Please. Don't move me."

"Okay," I said, stepping back. "I won't." I sure didn't want to hurt him, and I didn't want to piss off the nurses and doctors. I glanced at Kyle and Julia to see if my suggestion had irritated them. From what I'd seen, docs and nurses had a pecking order that was stricter than the fire department's. Once, at a fire scene, I'd made a suggestion which, in retrospect, was probably pretty arrogant since I was still a rookie at the time. "Fuck you, boy," one of the officers had said. "We don't pay you to think." He pointed to the canvas hose I held. "You just hump that hose." No one in the ER had been that blunt, but I didn't want to push my luck.

I looked at Mr. Meyers, his eyes closed, head tilted back into the pillow of the stretcher. His breathing was slower and deeper, but not natural. It was too regular, like he was aware of it. Mr. Meyers was still in pain.

"Foreshortened and externally rotated," Kyle said.

"Huh?" *Was he talking to me?* Since we wore scrubs just like the nurses and docs, the docs would sometimes forget that we were just nursing assistants, and explain stuff to us. It was as if the visual cues of our dress blurred the distinctions in our roles and status. I was flattered. Kyle seemed so far above me: his job was learning medicine and treating patients; my job was pushing stretchers, changing the sheets, and rinsing out bedpans. Kyle was what I hoped to become.

"Foreshortened and externally rotated," Kyle repeated. "See how his foot's pointing off to the side, and how that leg looks shorter than the other?"

I looked carefully from the patient's right foot to the left, then back.

Mr. Meyers grunted. Still hurting.

Kyle didn't seem to notice. "Little old ladies get the same thing when they break their hips. The muscles in the thigh pull the leg up and out to the side." He wrote something on the chart. "I'll give him a gram of Ancef, and some Gentamycin." The IV antibiotics would decrease the chance of an infection. Kyle walked toward the nurses' station.

I envied his casual confidence, but I wondered how he could seem so oblivious to the man's pain. I moved up to the head of the stretcher. "I hope you feel better soon," I said, having nothing else to offer.

Mr. Meyers opened his eyes to look at me and said, "Thanks." He closed his eyes again.

I backed away from the stretcher. Kyle had known exactly what to do: he'd given him morphine, antibiotics, checked the arteries and nerves, even marked the pulses so other people could check, too. He'd addressed every problem.

But damn, he'd seemed so callous. I wondered if he'd been like that before he started, or if medical school and internship had done it to him. And if med school could change people that much, did I really want to go? My Quaker parents had stressed the importance of caring about other people, which I thought required gentleness and a soft voice and an open heart.

A tech from the operating room came down to get the man with the bone angling out of his thigh. I helped push the stretcher down the hallway to the elevator. When the doors opened, the elevator floor was an inch lower than the hallway. I pulled back on the stretcher to decrease the jolting as the wheels bumped down across the threshold. Mr. Meyers winced, but didn't grunt or whimper. On the second floor, we eased out into the hallway with hardly a bump. He let out a deep breath, as we rolled him to the operating room. Signs on the double doors said, in large red lettering, NO ADMITTANCE.

"Thanks," the tech said. "I can take it from here." As he wheeled my guy through the doors, I longed for a more important role to play. Watching the doors swing shut, I knew that I wanted to be a doctor.

THE CARING CURVE

A COUPLE of years later, I was accepted into medical school at the University of North Carolina at Chapel Hill. We spent the first two years in classrooms and laboratories. In anatomy lab, we huddled around cadavers in groups of four. As a nursing assistant, I had helped wash the newly dead and wrap them in clean sheets before zipping them into thick, translucent bags. We would then heft the ungainly bundles onto special carts, and I would push them to the morgue. Since I had already handled corpses, I didn't expect the cadaver to bother me. But the first few times I lifted the damp cloth we kept draped over the leathery contours of his face, I avoided looking at the dried-out eyes that had shriveled back into their sockets.

Using saws, scalpels, and our fingers, we tried to create precise and elegant dissections from the dead bodies lying on stainless steel tables. In the color plates of *Clemente's Atlas of Human Anatomy*, the muscles were shown in striated reds and pinks, and the arteries were plump and full and a deep rich red. I imagined them pulsating with life and purpose. I loved the way the blue veins and yellow nerves ran gracefully and discretely alongside the arteries, beautiful in form and function.

But the tissue of our preserved corpse was brownish-gray and stringy, and the empty veins and arteries all looked the same. Somebody compared it to deboning the dried-out carcass of a Christmas turkey after it had been left on the counter overnight, and then taking an exam on what we'd seen.

In our dissecting group, two of us wanted to preserve the cadaver, and two of us were eager to cut it open and look inside. The preservationists moved with excruciating caution. They'd look at the pictures in the atlas, tug on a strand of tissue, look back at the book, scrape some of the crud off the nerve or artery or vein, then look back at the book. The other cutter or I would say, "Go ahead. Cut it." The guy was already dead, what difference could it make?

There was only room for two of our group to dissect at a time, so a couple of us would work with the scalpels, and the others would watch, make notes, and flip back and forth between several anatomy texts, looking for information that would help us decide if the stringy gray strand of tissue running beside the medial epicondyle of the elbow was the superior ulnar collateral artery, the ulnar nerve, the basilic vein, or just a strand of connective tissue we should've cut out of the way. Finally, I said, "Cut it and see if it's hollow inside."

A preservationist covered the desiccated bit of meat with a gloved hand, and said, "No. Wait." If they had their way, the anatomy session would be over before they'd cut through the first layer of skin. But if they hadn't insisted that the cutters exercise some caution, our cadaver would've looked like we had pushed it through a wood chipper. After the first few sessions, we paired up a preservationist and a cutter—giving each team someone to keep things moving, as well as someone to keep us from slashing off in the wrong direction.

The smell of formaldehyde leached through our gloves and into our skin. After anatomy lab we'd wash our hands over and over, trying to get the smell out. Someone brought in a can of "Beard Buster" shaving cream which upperclassmen had said cut the smell. But it didn't really. Just made our hands smell like a freshly shaved cadaver.

There was a crushing amount of detail to memorize in gross anatomy, but at least it was concrete and finite. Other classes—physiology, pathophysiology, histology—required massive amounts of detail, but you also had to *understand* it. One of my classmates said, "It's like trying to drink from a fire hydrant. You feel like you're going to explode from all the information you're taking in." I didn't tell her that as a firefighter I had drunk from a fire hydrant, and it wasn't that hard—you just had to turn it down until it was manageable. Of course, in medical school, there was no valve to turn down the flow.

You'd think that after being flooded with the Latin names in anatomy, the changing morphology of embryology, and the endless feedback loops of endocrinology, we would welcome some of the "softer" subjects. Instead, the lectures on medical ethics and seminars in medical humanities merely underscored our need for relief from the volume of work required. Many of us felt as if the professors were like the string quartet who played as the *Titanic* sank—"Thanks for the background music, fellas, but what I really want is a *lifeboat*."

One of our professors started his lecture with a question: "Who do you think was the most empathetic to the survivors of car wrecks that had involved fatalities?" The professor stood at the front of the classroom, his hands behind his back. "Was it the cop at the scene, the nurse in the ER, or the physician in the ER?" He raised his eyebrows and waited.

I knew it had to be the nurses.

"The cops." The professor chuckled and shook his head. "The cops were more caring than the nurses, who were more caring than the doctors."

So? I felt my face flush hot, as if I were already accused of callousness. Maybe the cops could seem more "caring" because it hadn't been their job to keep someone alive. Maybe the cops didn't have anything to do other than watch the firefighters hose down the spilled gasoline.

"The doctors had all slipped down the caring curve," the professor said. He then turned toward the blackboard and in a brisk, sweeping motion drew a curve in white chalk. He added in the vertical and horizontal lines representing the X and Y axes of a graph, and turned to face us again.

We were accustomed to seeing graphs, equations, and molecular structures chalked out in front of us, and most of us dutifully copied the diagram into our notebooks. The curve looked like a ski slope, which started at a level just above the professor's head and ran steeply downward to a level just below his waist, before scooping back up to the level of his chest. "Researchers took a cohort of premed students and gave them a test that would measure empathy and altruism, which they graphed on the Y axis." He scribbled the word "empathy" sideways, running up the Y axis. "The X axis represents time." He made a small mark at the top of the slope. "This point represents the premed responses." He then made a mark where the slope began to gradually trend downward. "The descent begins during the preclinical years, and accelerates as the medical students go through clinical rotations in the hospital. You can see that during residency, it plummets." He took his chalk and made a short slash across the graph at each transition. "Empathy bottoms out a few years after residency." He pointed at the upswing. "Empathy improves as clinicians get out in practice, but it never gets back to its initial value." He put the chalk down in the tray that ran the length of the blackboard, and dusted his fingers against his thumb.

The "caring curve" was interesting, but it seemed to me that compassion was something you should have learned before applying to medical school. And I was much more confident of my ability to remain compassionate than I was of mastering enough anatomy, biochemistry, pathophysiology—it went on and on—to keep from hurting someone out of ignorance. If a neurosurgeon seems brusque, a patient will tell his friends and family that his doc was uncaring. If a neurosurgeon isn't certain of the vascular supply to the cerebral cortex, the patient may not complain about anything.

Of course, you can become technically proficient and still care about people. But when your grasp of neuroanatomy is tenuous, and you're a little fuzzy on just how the circumflex branch of the left coronary artery wraps around the heart, you're scrambling too fast to fill the knowledge deficit to worry about your future bedside manner.

At the end of the second year, we all bought white coats. Forty percent polyester, they were stiff, and smelled of sizing. Each had a breast pocket, and two large patch pockets sewn to the front. We picked them up from the medical bookstore, a crowded little room packed floor-to-ceiling with textbooks, percussion hammers, stethoscopes—all the knickknackery of doctoring. My coat was baggy, and the sleeves seemed an inch too long. A classmate assured me that after I washed it, the fit would be perfect. We stuffed our pockets with the small spiral-ring reference booklets we hoped would bail us out if we forgot something, and draped our stethoscopes around our necks. The stethoscope was new and stiff and didn't drape comfortably or securely. I kept touching the head of the scope where it rested just above my right collarbone, afraid it would slip off in front of a patient, nurse, or doctor.

The bookstore opened up to a brick courtyard. If you turned right, you went back to the medical school; if you turned left, you walked into the hospital.

We were nervous, but excited. For two years we'd wanted to escape from the lecture halls and labs, and get to the hospital wards where we'd learn to take care of real patients with real problems: people who needed our help. Solving medical problems while at the same time showing compassion was no longer a lecture topic—it was for real. We would get on-the-job training.

"Never, ever," a professor would tell us, "let me hear you refer to a patient as 'The pneumonia in room four-one-five-five.'" Our small group of medical students and interns standing in the hallway outside a patient's room leaned closer to hear better. "You may have a patient with pneumonia, but she is much, much more than a disease process." The professor looked down at the floor, his chin spreading against his perfectly knotted tie, then looked up, making eye contact with each of us in turn. "Each patient is a person. While you are on *my* service, you'll treat them as such." Of course, he'd been right: People are individuals, with our own stories and relationships. His message resonated with my upbringing.

But in some emergencies, the last thing you want the doctor to do is consider you as a person. Years after I'd finished my internship and residency, I was the attending physician in an ER—the doctor in charge—when the paramedics brought in a drowned seven-year-old. The boy's wet blond hair fanned across his forehead as if he'd just climbed out of a pool. His lips were blue and his unmoving eyes stared up past long, wet lashes. His teeth rested against the plastic tube the paramedics had slipped down his windpipe. He looked like my son, John, and he was dead.

I was frozen by the enormity of what I faced.

"Paul," one of the nurses called.

"Continue CPR," I said reflexively to the nurse poised over the child's chest. I told myself to just do the drill. This small thing on my stretcher wasn't a child: he represented a series of decisions I had to make; an exercise the team and I had to go through. And any redemption we could pull from that room would be a function of how well we did our jobs. On some level, it didn't matter whether the small wet thing would become a child again or would be taken to the morgue: our only hope for solace would hinge on working quickly and efficiently. I packed my emotions down into a place where they wouldn't interfere.

After fifteen minutes of pumping on his chest, squeezing air into his lungs, and pushing medications into his bloodstream, we finally got a pulse back. No one cheered, or even smiled. We were just doing a drill, and knew we could lose the pulse at any time. A paramedic came into the room and said that the boy's dad had shown up. The paramedic gestured to the child on the stretcher and lowered his voice. "We found him in his dad's girlfriend's backyard swimming pool. The mom's on the way."

"His dad's *girlfriend's* pool?" Of all the places a kid could drown. I shook my head. I took a deep breath and exhaled through pursed lips. With the immediate crisis stabilized, my emotions began to stir. I had to clamp them down again. It was time to talk with the boy's father, a man I'd never met and would never see again.

He was pale. His lips trembled. He kept his eyes focused on the floor. I told him, in a clear and calm voice, that we'd gotten the boy's heart beating again and that a machine was breathing for him. I told him we'd transfer him to the university medical center across town, where they had a pediatric intensive care unit. The man looked up to my eyes, then back to the floor. I told him I didn't know when, or if, the boy would start breathing on his own. I didn't know if he'd regain consciousness. The man wiped his cheek with the back of his hand.

What I didn't tell him was that I, too, had a son, with blond hair and long eyelashes. I didn't tell him I'd been terrified of failing, or that I, too, felt like crying. My feelings were small and unimportant in the presence of a man standing at the edge of such vast loss and guilt. And I didn't have time for feelings; the ER was filled with other patients, and I had six more hours to work. The best I could do for the boy's father was to give him room, and offer a gentle and steady presence. Emotional distance may not always indicate a failure of empathy—giving the boy's father a respectful space may have been the most compassionate thing I could've done.

SOMETHING SO PERSONAL

"So," Dr. Jameson said, his hand loosely holding the steering wheel of his Mercedes. "Tell me about your family." He glanced to the left, then right, and pulled out of the parking lot of his office. Dr. Jameson was a surgeon in a small town in North Carolina, with a clinical appointment at UNC.

I was a fourth-year medical student, and had been paired with him for a rotation in general surgery. It was time for me to choose which specialty I wanted to go into. I'd enjoyed surgery, but after five years on the fire department, and two years working in the ER as an undergraduate, emergency medicine seemed like a good fit, too. This rotation would be the tie-breaker.

"Sally, my wife, is a nurse," I said. "Right now, she's taking time off to be with our daughter, Sarah. She's one year old."

The leather seat of the car was hot from baking in the afternoon sun, so I sat forward. Dr. Jameson had turned on the air conditioner, but hadn't rolled down the windows.

"It's good your wife is staying home with the baby. There's no substitute for a mother in the home." He looked at me, nodded, then looked back to the road. "People will blather on about the virtues of day care," he said, "but they're wrong."

I'd been working with Dr. Jameson for about a week. Born and raised in Cape Town, South Africa, he'd trained in England. "I'm a Fellow in the Royal Academy of Surgeons," he'd told me, in a subtle British accent. A heavy man, he stood with perfect posture; his head tilted just about half a degree back. He was usually pleasant, polite, and precise in his speech.

"I'm really glad that Sally wants to be a full-time mom," I said. "Sarah has Down syndrome, so she needs all the help she can get." I felt sweat run from my armpit, down my side, inside my shirt.

"Down syndrome?" His voice was quiet. "So sorry." His eyes moved to the rearview mirror, and he changed lanes. We drove in silence for half a block. "The only thing to do," he said crisply, "is put her in an institution." He made a brisk chopping motion with his right hand. "It would hurt for a couple of weeks, maybe a couple of months. But better to have that one searing moment of pain, and then move on with your life." He nodded to himself. "Start over."

I sat still, gazing through the windshield at the back of the pickup truck in front of us. Even factoring in cultural differences, and the fact he was an attending and I was just a medical student, I was stunned he'd say something so personal.

Of course, I'd been the one to bring up Down syndrome. But I've never known what to do about telling people. It's not something I have to confess to everyone I meet, but I like to let people know. When I was twenty-three, working on the fire department, I was talking with a guy from another fire station who had a baby. "I bet you've been busy, with a curtain climber in the house," I said, with nothing better to say. "He's not a *curtain climber*." The man scowled, and turned away. I found out later that his kid had cerebral palsy.

"Everyone says Down syndromes are loving." Dr. Jameson shrugged. "And they are, after a fashion." He glanced over at me, then back to the road. "But they'll love you without reservation one day, and you'll be a total stranger the very next." He shook his head. "Forgive me for my bluntness, but that is my advice." He made another chopping motion with his right hand. "Take her somewhere, leave her with competent people, and start over."

I had the feeling that if we passed an institution for the mentally infirm, he'd stop, walk in with me, and get me started on the paperwork.

I sat, trying to think of something to say that wouldn't fuck up my grade. He seemed oblivious to how offensive his advice had been. Maybe in Cape Town, or London, they talked that way.

I looked out the window. Of course, it's not like it hadn't occurred to me, and the idea had a guilty appeal. But Sally and I had discussed it, and she felt very strongly that we should keep Sarah. If I was going to have one searing moment of pain, it would involve the loss of my wife as well as my daughter.

I COULDN'T IMAGINE splitting up with Sally. I'd met her five years previously, at an ER Christmas party. She'd come with a friend of mine named Dylan. He was an older college student like me, working part time in the emergency room. When Dylan introduced us, Sally smiled, her eyes crinkling at the corners. Her hair, parted at the middle, flowed out past her shoulders in a wild and churning mass of curls. She batted it back, and stuck out her hand. "Nice to meet you." Her handshake was firm and brisk. Her jaw was square at the angle, delicately prominent. Sally stood straight, shoulders back, relaxed but taut. I'd thought of Katharine Hepburn in *The African Queen*, and wondered if Dylan's girlfriend was as restrained, and as classy, as Hepburn. Okay, probably not as tightly wound as Hepburn's character. Sally wore low-riding jeans, scuffed brown clogs, and a black Danskin top, without a bra.

I liked being near this smart woman with the unabashedly southern accent. She swayed subtly with the music as she stood and talked, and I envied Dylan. The next day, at work, he told me they were just friends.

A few months later, Dylan invited each of us to his birthday party so we could meet. I got off work that night at eleven, stripped off my scrubs and put on some jeans, and went to Dylan's house. Sally was as compelling as I'd remembered, and I was surprised at how relaxed I felt talking with her. Her eyes were gray-blue, with a thin rim of gold surrounding the pupils. When she laughed, her eyes became merry slits. I was afraid I'd been telling too many stories, so I made myself shut up, to give her a chance to talk. She worked as a psychiatric nurse, on a locked ward—adolescents who'd been involuntarily committed. When working the night shift, she had to check every patient every fifteen minutes. She'd tiptoe into their room with a narrow-beam flashlight, to make sure they were still breathing. "You watch for the rise and fall of their chests." At first she'd felt intrusive, slipping into such private spaces, watching for the rustling movements of troubled dreams, listening to the snuffling sounds of sleep. She didn't like doing it, but understood why the requirement existed. "If somebody's really determined, they can kill themselves even on a locked ward. You don't want the day shift to come in, pull down the covers, and find a cold body." Other routines seemed just as exotic and mundane. Each morning they'd make the anorexic girls void their bladders before the morning weigh-in. "Otherwise they'd store up urine all night to get credit for gaining a few ounces of weight they could then just flush down the toilet."

Sally had gotten her master's degree in nursing in Gainesville, Florida, specializing in eating disorders and adolescent psychiatry. "I love that age group. They have so much energy, and they can still change."

I'd gone to the party with the goal of meeting Sally. Having done so, I wanted to leave because I had to be at work the next morning at seven o'clock. Sally left with me. We stood beside her car, a metallic green Mustang. She must've heard "Mustang Sally" a hundred times so I didn't mention it.

"I'd like to see you again," I said. My calendar, which I always carried in my back pocket, had a color-coded system to keep my life straight: my shifts in the ER were in blue ink, my classes in black, paydays in green, and exams in red. I was afraid it would expose me as hopelessly uncool and obsessive, so I didn't pull it out.

The next day I called her, and invited her to dinner at my house—a single-wide mobile home outside of Chapel Hill. I baked a quiche because it seemed sophisticated, and because I was proud that I could make a decent pie crust from scratch. I bought two wineglasses and a bottle of Chablis. Afraid I'd be clumsy with the cork, I pulled it out with my Swiss army knife before she arrived.

Sally brought daffodils wrapped in a cone of newspaper, and asked for a knife to trim each stem. "Makes 'em last longer," she said, slipping a flower into the water glass I'd filled. "The capillary action doesn't work as well when the ends are dried out."

Made sense.

"Don't you love the physics of things?" she asked.

I stared at her back, the lines of her shoulder blades angular through the thin knit cotton of her turtleneck, her narrow waist, and the worn white ovals on the seat of her jeans. "Yes," I said. "I do."

During supper, I told some stories from my dropout years. Eventually I worked around to my marriage and separation from Barbara, my wife of five years who'd left me six months earlier. "She thought I worked and studied too much."

"And?" Sally took a sip of wine.

"Said I was too intense."

Sally laughed. "I meant, did you think she was right about working and studying?"

"Probably." I ate a bite of quiche. "But you can't get into med school without studying your ass off. At least I can't." I was ready to get off the hot seat. "Dylan said you've never been married."

She coughed, and smoothed her napkin in her lap. "I'm in analysis now, trying to figure out why none of my relationships has ever worked out."

I nodded, but I'd never been sure psychiatry was for real. I wanted to be a surgeon, or an ER doc—actually do something other than listen to people chatter endlessly about their problems.

After a silence that seemed amiable, Sally asked me about school. I told her I was a zoology major—biology without the plants.

"Premed?"

"We'll see." I gave her my stock answer. "If I get in, I'll have been premed. If I don't get in, I'll have been pre-something else."

"And if you don't?"

"I'll keep trying."

When we finished the wine, Sally said it was time to go. I walked her to her car, where she stopped and turned her face up to mine. I leaned down and paused. She moved toward me, and we kissed briefly, then pulled away. She put her arms around my waist and we kissed again, longer. "What are we doing here?" I said. I hoped she'd want to stay over.

"We're saying good night." She kissed me again. "Thanks for a wonderful dinner."

On our next date, Sally took me for a walk along the Eno River. She wore faded jeans, a crimson ski jacket, and brown leather hiking boots with thick red laces. As we walked side by side, I wanted to reach over to hold her hand, but was afraid it would make me seem like a nervous junior high school kid.

"The redbuds are almost out." Sally paused and held back a thin branch that had been arcing across the trail. "See?" She brushed her fingertips across the hard purple nubs sprouting from the limb.

I looked closely at her fingernails, unpolished and short, her hands, clean and competent. I wondered whether the curve of her neck would smell like soap. We walked until we came to a spot where water-smoothed stones led to a large, flat rock in the middle of the river.

"I should tell you that I'm not looking for casual sex," she said, stepping from the bank onto a rock, and then skipping to one further out.

I stepped onto the rock she'd just left. "What kind of sex are you looking for?"

She laughed. "You know what I mean." She looked at me. "I've always settled for short-term affairs that weren't going anywhere.

I'm tired of that." She took two quick steps onto rocks further in the stream. "If you're not interested in a real relationship, I'd rather know it now," she called over her shoulder.

"I'm not afraid of commitment . . . " I stepped to a rock closer to hers.

"But . . . " Sally stopped, turned, and put her hands on her hips.

I shrugged. "Maybe I should sign some divorce papers before we start discussing china patterns."

She laughed again. "Good point." She shaded her eyes with her hand. "I know it's too soon to talk about commitments. I just don't want to start another relationship if I know in advance it's is going to be a dead end."

"Fair enough." I looked down the river to an outcropping of rocks that had snagged a tree limb as it floated downstream. A lost fisherman's line with its red-and-white bobber was tangled in the branches. After Barbara had left, I'd ricocheted through a couple of very brief relationships, and had begun to feel lonesome. I stepped onto the stone next to hers. My rock teetered side to side.

"This is an new experience for me," she said. "Saying, up front, what I'm looking for."

"Me too." I felt as if we were prearranging a business agreement, or working on a treaty between two sovereign states. I looked again at the water flowing through the snag downstream, then back to Sally.

"And?" She looked me in the eyes. She had to squint because of the sun reflecting off of the water.

"We'll have to see where it goes. Maybe short term, hopefully long term."

"Fair enough." Her hands were resting on her hips.

I wondered if I should reach out to shake hands on the deal, but she was on her rock and I was on mine. Mine was feeling wobbly.

As a staff nurse on psychiatry, Sally had to work her share of night shifts and weekends, so we had to juggle our schedules to spend time together. Our dates were typically inexpensive—a free movie at the student union, and then a couple of beers at He's Not Here, a bar on Franklin Street. One night we lay on our backs in the middle of a fairway on the Duke Golf Course, watching for meteors. We hadn't seen any. "There's Venus," she said, pointing about thirty degrees up from the horizon. "See it?"

"I'm not sure." I moved closer to sight down her arm.

"It's the one that's not twinkling." Sally had taken astronomy as an undergraduate, and could still pick out the planets and constellations. I was impressed that she could remember so much of what she'd learned, but I couldn't imagine taking astronomy unless I planned to make a career of it. I turned to look at her profile. "How did you end up in that class?"

"I was interested in it." She looked over to me. "Why?"

I shrugged in the dark. "Just curious." I looked back up to the black and glittering sky. Sally seemed interested in almost everything around her, whether it was trees, stars, or human behavior. She enjoyed strolling through the Ackland Art Museum, Nice Price Books, and Huggins Hardware Store. This same woman who skied in Aspen didn't hesitate to put her hands in the dirt to help plant tomatoes and daffodils in front of my mobile home. And she seemed so calm. I was drawn to that.

"Show me Venus again."

* * *

During a spring break, we drove Sally's Mustang down to Key West. Twenty-four hours straight through, we took turns driving, cat-napping, and helping each other stay awake.

Two of my professors had scheduled exams during the first week after spring break, so I knew I'd have to study while we were in Key West. I got up every morning at six o'clock, and slipped out to a little place that served Cuban coffee and huevos rancheros. That early in the morning most of the other customers were tradesmen, stopping by on the way to work. I enjoyed quizzing myself and flipping through my notecards as I ate breakfast with the locals.

By ten, I'd studied enough not to feel guilty for taking the rest of the day off. Sally would have gotten up and had a cup of coffee and a muffin, and we could spend the rest of the day together—walking on the beach or dozing in the sun. At night, her skin smelled of coconut oil. I was surprised at how easily and naturally things worked out when I was with her.

Six months later, we went to a party in Chapel Hill. I'd just pulled off the asphalt onto the grass at the side of the road. Sally unbuckled her seatbelt. "I think it's time we decided where we're going."

"To your friend's birthday?" I gestured with my chin toward the yellow light and laughter coming through the screen windows.

"No," Sally said. "As a couple." She shifted in the MG's bucket seat to face me. "I'm ready to get married."

"Okay."

"Okay?" Sally leaned forward to look me in the eyes. "That's it?"

"We're past the point of me getting down on one knee, don't you think?"

"Were you planning to?"

"Well, yeah," I said. "After I get into medical school."

"I've always hoped to get married by the time I turn thirty." Sally sat back in her seat, facing forward.

Neither of us had highly romanticized notions about marriage. Sally's father, a psychiatrist, had always told her that the idea of "one perfect match" only holds true in romance novels. In real life, you will meet multiple people who would make a suitable mate. His advice was to find someone who's compatible, marry him, and expect that you both will have to work at it. Sally was a practical woman, and as a nurse she had seen doctors-in-training at their best and worst—hardworking and caring, but also sleep-deprived, and sometimes petulant. She felt that she knew what she was getting into.

We were sitting shoulder to shoulder in the car's snug interior, each looking straight ahead through the windshield. Another couple walked past holding hands. They waved to us and smiled. We waved back.

I'd never been loved by a woman as smart, good-looking, and even-tempered as Sally. Even so, I was in no rush to get married. After witnessing my parents' divorce and experiencing my own, marriage seemed like a huge and unpredictable gamble. Getting married again would risk the possibility of failing twice. But then I considered the risk she was taking with me—a part-time nursing assistant living in a mobile home with green shag carpet. Who was I to balk? I turned toward her. "We don't have to wait."

She thought a minute. "Okay." She opened her door and climbed out.

I got out my side and looked at her over the canvas car roof. "So, we're engaged?"

"You tell me."

I stuck out my bottom lip and raised my eyebrows. "I'd say so."

We walked toward the party, holding hands. Inside, I listened to see if Sally would mention it to any of her friends, but she didn't. On the drive to her apartment, I asked her if she felt different.

"Not so far," she said.

"Me neither."

We were married August 11, 1984, in an outdoor theater on the campus of the University of North Carolina in Chapel Hill. A string quartet played as our guests walked in. Sally wore white, and I wore a light gray suit and a red silk tie. Sally's mother hosted the reception in their backyard, a smooth expanse of grass, trees, and azaleas, backing up to a lake. Relaxed, but classy. I felt like I was marrying into a family that understood how to enjoy themselves, and I hoped to get the hang of it myself.

My only misgiving had been her background: Sally didn't seem to think it remarkable that she'd gone to high school at Holton Arms, a D.C. boarding school for the daughters of senators and the future brides of presidents. Sally's parents knew how to order wine in restaurants, and her entire family knew how to snow-ski. I'd left home at nineteen, and felt that my only hope of happiness would be the product of relentless effort. I was afraid that Sally's life had been too sheltered to prepare her for any real problems, and if we encountered any heavy weather she'd just peel away like the roof of a mobile home in a hurricane. But when Sarah was born, Sally proved tougher and braver than I did.

As the obstetrician pulled our baby's slippery body out from Sally's, no lusty cry greeted us. No clenched little fists protested the cold dry air. The newborn's eyes were slanted and her body was slow and floppy. Dr. Nicholson said our baby had Down syndrome. He spoke softly, gently, and clearly. He told us that the baby's heart had a small defect, an abnormal window between two chambers, allowing fresh blood to mix with stale.

I saw a ray of hope—maybe the defect would be fatal and we could bury this mistake. Start over, after the tears had dried. I was ashamed of such an ugly wish, but Down syndrome, so aptly named, was a problem other people had. Fathers different from me: unlucky men who'd been singled out, as if God had leaned down and put his thumb in the center of their foreheads and applied enough pressure to mark them as the unfortunate souls they were—just in case you couldn't already tell from their kid's electric wheelchairs, or the padded helmets they wore.

Dr. Nicholson waited.

Sally was quiet for several seconds, and then began to scream. With each gasp, a vein snaked across her forehead. Her hair was stringy with sweat. She held her arms tight against her body. Her fists were hard, angry knots. Married for five years, I'd heard her cry, and sometimes curse, but never shriek. Was she howling for the normal baby who'd failed to surface, or was it the hole in this baby's heart? I didn't know if she feared the death of this baby, or if she shared my guilty hope. Stunned, I held her hand, wondering why I wasn't crying, too. Finally, Sally stopped crying. I handed her a Kleenex.

"Thanks." She snuffled, and tried to smile. Shaking her head, she started sobbing again.

I leaned over to kiss the top of her head. I held the position until my back cramped from leaning over the side rails of her bed. I slid a chair over next to her bed.

She looked at me and slowly shook her head.

"Buddy," I whispered, "I'm sorry."

She nodded. "Me, too." Her face knotted up again. Slowly the crying stopped. Sally lay with her eyes shut.

"Have you chosen a name?" Dr. Nicholson asked.

I looked at Sally. We had decided on Sarah, but I wasn't sure we wanted to use such a pretty name on this baby who was so very different from what we'd expected.

"Sarah." Sally kept her eyes closed. "We will call her Sarah." Her voice was hoarse, but clear.

DR. JAMESON REACHED forward and turned on the radio, preset to a classical station. I glanced at him, expecting him to repeat his advice to dump my daughter. I looked back out the window.

When I was fifteen, I'd visited an institution for people with mental and emotional disabilities. I'd been working through the summer as a dishwasher at Quaker Lake Camp, and they took us on field trips to see opportunities for helping less fortunate people. A kid whose eyes were too close together sat alone, hugging herself and rocking front to back. She'd glance up at us, then back to her lap. Another girl walked right up to me and grabbed my hand. Her fingers were sticky, and she stood too close.

The nurses tricked the girls into taking their medication by putting the pills in spoonfuls of applesauce. "Snack time," the nurse said, to the slope-eyed, grinning girl. The girl opened her mouth. "You like applesauce, don't you?" She sounded like she was talking to a baby, or a dog, or a parakeet. The nurse slipped the spoon into the girl's mouth. The girl closed her lips, and the spoon came out clean. "Good girl," the nurse said.

Even if Sally agreed, how could I park my car, set the emergency brake, and carry Sarah into a place smelling of Clorox and stale piss? And how could I walk away? Would we go back to visit her on her birthday, and at Christmas?

As I sat in Dr. Jameson's car, wishing the air conditioning would cool off sooner, I imagined a life that didn't include a daughter with Down syndrome. I imagined flipping through a photo album—in one picture, Sally and I would stand in hiking gear with our arms draped over the shoulders of two healthy kids, with the Appalachian Trail receding up into the background. On another page, the same two kids would shade their eyes as they grinned up at the camera from behind a sandcastle surrounded by shell-encrusted turrets. A family in which the children were all normal.

Dr. Jameson pulled into the hospital parking lot. "This close enough?" he asked.

"Sure," I said. "Our building is just over there." I pointed to the white stucco building twenty-five yards away, in the shadows of a thick grove of pine trees. "Thanks." I got out of his car.

"Best of luck with your . . ." He cleared his throat. "With your difficulties."

I leaned over to look at him.

He ducked his head, as if embarrassed, or pained.

"Thanks," I said again, closing the door. I turned and walked toward our student apartment, a dark place with a subtle moldy smell. I heard Dr. Jameson's car pull away.

His suggestion had unsettled me, and I didn't feel ready to face my wife, or daughter. After five years of marriage, I loved Sally, and liked her, more than ever. I liked the way she woke up in the mornings; still sleepy, but glad to see me. I liked the small beads of sweat in her hairline when she came home from her modern dance class. I liked the way she read different novels from me. I liked sharing the paper with her during breakfast, reading the comics while she read the front page, and then switching. I liked the calm intelligence in her eyes.

The year before, while rotating through a pediatric oncology ward, I'd seen a girl who looked to be about five years old. She wore a child's patient gown, printed with blue, red, and yellow balloons. Her bald head perched delicately on her thin, knobby neck. With her left hand, she pushed a rolling IV pole. Clear tubing snaked from the bag of fluid, gently swinging side to side in cadence with her short steps. Her right hand clasped her mom's. Halfway down the hall they stopped, walked into a room, and closed the door.

I stood with the residents and the attending physician, in a cluster of white coats. "How do the parents do it?" I had asked the attending.

He'd nodded that he understood my question. "The strong families come together," he said in a quiet tone. He shrugged one shoulder. "The weaker couples split up." He looked to the floor, then back to me. "It's hard."

I glanced back to where Dr. Jameson had dropped me off, then stepped onto the concrete porch of the student housing building. I stared at the brown metal door and took a deep breath. I let out the breath, turned the key in the lock, and stepped into the cool, dark room. I moved carefully and quietly, in case our daughter was down for a nap.

DECLARING A PATIENT

"THIS is the medicine intern," I said into the phone, "returning a page." I turned on the lamp on the table next to my bed and squinted at my watch: 4:30 in the morning. I'd slept about an hour and a half. Not too bad, since I'd caught a couple of hours of sleep earlier in the night.

"You need to come declare a patient." I didn't recognize the voice. I was in my second month of a rotating internship in emergency medicine at one of the biggest hospitals in Pittsburgh: seven hundred beds and twenty-eight hundred nurses.

"Declare?" I yawned.

"Dead," she answered. I heard someone in the background chuckle.

"What?" I shielded my eyes against the light, feeling sleepy and dim-witted.

"You need to declare a patient dead." Her tone flattened.

"Oh, okay," I said. "I'll be right there." We hung up. At that time of the morning my mind was a blunt instrument, so I was glad it was something simple, instead of a patient with acute chest pain, or shortness of breath, or some other problem I'd have to really think about.

I'd been in the hospital since six the previous morning, and wouldn't go home until my work was done later that day, hopefully by five or six in the evening. Sally was a nurse and had seen what internship was like, so she'd forgive me for wolfing down supper and dropping straight into bed. But if I could knock out this problem and rack up another hour of sleep, I'd have enough reserve to stay up for an hour or so when I got home. I wanted to reconnect with Sally and play with Sarah, who by then had turned three years old.

I was doing a residency in emergency medicine rather than surgery, even though I'd always enjoyed working with my hands. Whether it was shaving off a thin curl of wood with a chisel, or getting a nut to thread on the bolt behind the starter of my MG, my hands seemed to understand things quickly. I'd worked diligently on my surgical rotations as a medical student, and knew I'd get good recommendations from the faculty. But I'd done poorly on the written exam, and finished the rotation with a pass instead of honors. Essentially, I'd made a C. The chairman of the department, Dr. Parini, called me into his office. "Paul, your grades on the clinical part of your rotation were excellent."

I nodded.

He opened a file folder on his desk and read out loud: "Outstanding . . . Good work ethic . . . positive attitude . . . takes excellent care of his patients . . . shows keen interest in OR." Dr. Parini glanced back down at the file on his desk. "But you almost failed the written exam."

I nodded again. I knew I hadn't studied enough. The book of practice questions my classmates had purchased in the medical bookstore had seemed less important than reviewing the anatomy for the cases I'd scrubbed in on, and I hadn't expected the exam to be that hard.

"I understand that you've recently had some difficulties with your family . . ."

"I've tried not to let it interfere." I sat straighter, feeling my face blush hot. I hoped I wasn't in trouble, but I sure as shit wasn't going to apologize for having a daughter with Down syndrome.

"No," he said, shaking his head. "That's not what I'm getting at. You've done well on your clinical rotation. But having a child with," he looked back to the papers in front of him, "a child with Down syndrome, that's bound to affect you." He looked up at me. "And it's why I've asked you to come by. I think you'd make a good surgeon."

"Thank you."

"We rarely do this." He paused. "But if you'd like, you can retake the written exam." He was giving me a second chance.

"Thank you, sir." The idea of becoming a surgeon had appeal, but I didn't want to squeak by on a second chance I'd been granted because my daughter had Down syndrome. I'd gotten into medical school by studying my ass off, grubbing for grades, and never missing a chance to get ahead. Surgery programs seemed to be the quintessential manifestation of that culture. Some surgery programs even had a pyramid system, in which there are fewer spots for the last years of residency than there are for the first year, requiring that every year a resident gets "cut," after finishing just a portion of his or her training. Retaking the exam based on family problems seemed like a sign of weakness, and surgery seemed the one specialty in which signs of weakness wouldn't be tolerated. "I appreciate your offer, but I think I'll stick with the grade I got."

"Okay." He closed the file folder and leaned back in his chair. "Your decision."

I'd been thinking about going into emergency medicine anyway. From what I'd seen, the ER docs just seemed happier than surgeons. Cooler, too. Maybe it's because they had more time off, or maybe it's because their work was more varied. And I'd felt drawn to the idea of being an all-round doc.

I yawned, and swung my feet off the bed. The on-call room was small and plain, about six feet by ten. The bare walls were painted eggshell white. A wooden chair sat at the foot of my bed, a Formica nightstand at the head. My white coat and stethoscope hung from a hook on the door. If Red Roof Inn were to design a monastery, my call room would be the result.

Had the nurse told me where I was supposed to go? I mean, where was the dead guy? And whose patient was he? Was he one of mine? *Damn.* I pushed the button on my beeper to show the last page received, and quickly punched the number into the phone. "Seven-one," the ward clerk answered, identifying the floor and unit she was working on.

"Do you-all have someone who needs to be declared?"

"What?" She didn't sound irritated, just confused.

"Did someone just page me to come declare a patient dead?"

"I'll check." She muffled the phone with her hand, and then came back. "Yeah. Mr. Brooks, room seven-oh-three."

I hung up. Not one of mine. Good.

I'd never declared anyone dead and had never seen it done. I got out my *Scut Monkey's Manual*, a chunky spiral-bound handbook that tells you how to do most of the tasks a medical student or intern has to do. SCUT stands for Some Common Unfinished Task, reflecting the countless unglamorous details that dominate a medical student or intern's life. In the section dedicated to chartwork, there were examples of a delivery note, a pre-op note, an operative note, and a problem-oriented progress note. But there was no information on declaring a patient dead, or the paperwork involved. I'd have to wing it; but how hard could it be, compared to the other things I'd done since graduating from medical school?

I expected internship to be stressful, and it was. On most rotations we were on call every third night, which wasn't too bad. Sometimes we were on every other, and would have to work thirty-six hours, catching sleep when we could. Our mantra was, "Eat when you can eat, sleep when you can sleep." I quickly learned from the senior residents to sneak off to a call room every chance I got, no matter what time of day. I would lie on my back and carefully smooth my hair under my head so I wouldn't get "bed head." Since my face wasn't pressed into the pillow, I never had the telltale pink wrinkles across my cheek or forehead. I can still sleep that way, flat on my back, arms to my sides. Snagging a thirty-minute nap in the afternoon was the mark of an efficient and savvy resident. Catching a few hours of sleep every night meant that you were good at getting your work done.

Residents are now limited to working eighty hours a week. The Accreditation Council for Graduate Medical Education made the decision in 2003, after a protracted national debate. A young doctor was quoted in *American Family Physician*, the journal of the American Academy of Family Physicians: "As a resident, it becomes exceptionally difficult to put forth the same amount of thought and offer the same emotional support to patients after a long 36-hour shift. The most disheartening feeling as a resident physician is when you feel that your own patients have become the enemy. By enemy, I mean the one thing that stands between you and a few hours of sleep." This quote was offered in support of stricter limits on resident hours. Taken at face value, there's little room for argument. But I wonder how doctors will learn to take care of patients when their empathy has been exhausted if they don't learn to do it in residency. Unless people are only going to get sick between nine and five, Monday through Friday, somebody's going to have to do some late night doctoring, even when they don't feel like it.

Across the country, hospitals are having difficulty finding specialists who are willing to be on call for emergencies. How many people would volunteer to climb out of bed at three o'clock in the morning to come into the ER to take care of a stranger, for free? In my hospital, just like hospitals across the country, the neurologists dropped their admitting privileges so they wouldn't have to take call. They no longer come to the ER to help decide if a patient having a stroke should be given TPA, the "clot buster medicine." That's not a trivial question, since 3 percent to 6 percent of the stroke patients who get thrombolytics will have fatal hemorrhage into their brain. It has happened to one of my patients. An elderly lady came into the ER having a stroke. I discussed it with a neurologist over the phone, reviewed the risks and benefits with her husband, and gave her the TPA. A short time later, her blood pressure skyrocketed and her respirations became erratic gasps. I stuck a plastic tube down her windpipe and got another CT scan of her brain. I helped push the woman's stretcher to the scanner, knowing she'd hemorrhaged inside the brain, but irrationally hoping she hadn't. I stood behind the CT tech and watched as the computer screen flashed up the pictures of the ugly clots of blood blossoming inside the woman's brain. If a neurologist *had* come in, I'm fairly sure that the same decisions would've been made, but we'll never know.

Friends outside of medicine have suggested that working long hours was simply a form of hazing that the old doctors perpetuated—"I went through it, so you'll have to as well." But as I was pulling my call in residency, it seemed that working through the night to help sick people was just another part of becoming a doctor.

I adapted to the call schedule; but I never got over the feeling of shame for not knowing more. Nights on call exposed the things I hadn't yet learned, things for which one couldn't really study: how many units of blood to transfuse into a person with a gastrointestinal bleed? What's the dose of a given antibiotic for a patient in kidney failure? How much oxygen should I give an elderly man with pneumonia?

Everyone realized that interns and residents were in the process of learning. That's why we were there. But nurses, patients, and families all seemed to think the intern already *knew* what he or she was supposed to be learning. And not knowing what to do while a person is gasping, moaning, or pissing blood is a discouraging experience. That, not the long hours, was to me the most stressful aspect of residency training. I think that's why so few people stop at car wrecks. Is there anything more miserable than standing in the presence of human suffering and not knowing what to do?

But after answering the page, I wasn't worried. I wouldn't have to make any important decisions, and I wouldn't need to wake up Shannon Rogerson, my senior resident. I could just tell her at sign-out rounds in the morning. The culture of the hospital ward was, "Call your senior if you have to, but *only* if you have to." If I called for help with every single problem that came up, the senior wouldn't get any sleep, and I wouldn't learn to think independently. Of course, whether or not I'd call depended on the personality of my senior as well as their specialty. As an ER resident rotating through the major specialties, I'd learned that the surgery seniors wanted to know of every potential problem as soon as possible, but got pissed if you hadn't thought of a solution before you called. Medicine residents, on the other hand, seemed to enjoy working out the details of a medical puzzle, and wanted to participate in every step of the decision-making process. In this case, it wasn't an issue; the nurse had already determined the guy was dead. My role was just a formality. I'd go upstairs, knock out the paperwork, and get back to my bed as quickly as possible.

I'd already learned that the hospital offered an almost endless pool of suffering, and if I was going to get through it intact, I'd have to limit how much of it I internalized. Maybe I had already started slipping down the "caring curve" our professor had drawn up on the blackboard back in the second year of medical school. It didn't seem like it at the time—it felt as if I'd just learned to be a more cautious investor of my emotions.

Not surprisingly, medical educators have written about this. In the journal *Academic Medicine*, Jack Coulehan, M.D., M.P.H., and Peter Williams, J.D., Ph.D., published "Vanishing Virtue: The Impact of Medical Education" in June 2001. They pointed out that medical schools actually teach two sets of values, each of which is divergent from the other. The first set, to which there is an *explicit* commitment, includes the traditional values of doctoring—empathy, compassion, and altruism. The second set, to which there is a *tacit* commitment, includes an ethic of detachment, self-interest, and objectivity. These divergent values (empathy, compassion, and altruism vs. detachment, self-interest, and objectivity) can be confusing to physicians-in-training. Some of these young physicians resolve the conflict by rationalizing that they best serve their patients by concentrating exclusively on technical competence. Coulehan and Williams suggest that more classes in family medicine, communication skills, medical ethics, humanities, and social issues in medicine would help.

Maybe they're right—maybe modern American medical education is producing crop after crop of uncaring physicians, and more classes would help. Perhaps traditional Chinese physicians are uniformly compassionate, but I bet after a long day of twisting needles into the skin of complaining, harping, miserable people, even they get a little testy.

Coulehan and Williams suggest that some young physicians may be immune to developing detachment, self-interest, and objectivity, and therefore more likely to hold to the traditional values of empathy, compassion, and altruism. This "immunization" could take the form of being a woman, having a strong personal belief system, or prior experience as a Peace Corps Volunteer or teaching in low-income-area schools. Maybe that is true—maybe non-traditional people are "immunized" against a loss of their compassion as they toil their way through medical training.

If that's the case, I was in great shape as a non-traditional intern. In junior high school I read every biography I could find about my heroes: Mahatma Gandhi, Henry David Thoreau, and Dr. Martin Luther King, Jr. I spent my summers volunteering full time in a Head Start center. Every Saturday morning I spent an hour in a silent vigil for peace in Vietnam.

Non-traditional? In high school I drove a school bus to pay

for a parcel of land in rural North Carolina. I dropped out of college to build a cabin on the land, and then went on to work as a pizza cook, trash truck laborer, and firefighter. If Coulehan and Williams were right, I should be fully immunized against any loss of compassion.

But at the time, I wasn't worrying about any of this stuff. Emotional distance seemed like the only sane response to the burden of suffering I saw. My plan was to save up my energy, fill the gaps in my fund of medical knowledge, and sleep every chance I got.

I scratched my head, and yawned. My mouth was thick with the stale taste of having slept with my mouth open, so I walked down a short hallway to the bathroom, splashed my face, and brushed my teeth. Some interns wanted everyone to know when they'd been up all night, suffering. Not me. I always shaved and showered, and put on clean underwear and socks, first thing in the morning after being on call.

Riding up in the elevator, I wondered about the term "declaring" a patient dead. Why not "say," (or "announce," or "confirm," or "assert") that someone has died? The elevator stopped, the doors slid open, and I walked down the hall until I got to room 703.

The door stood ajar. I paused, and then tiptoed into the dimly lit room. I'd helped care for dead bodies as a nursing assistant, and had dissected one as a medical student, but being alone in a room with a dead person still made me uneasy. My eyes adjusted, and I could see well enough. An old man lay on the bed, the sheets folded neatly down just below his chest. He had white hair, parted on the side, not combed, but not particularly mussed.

I glanced around the room, unsure how to begin. In CPR

classes we had been taught to firmly tap the mannequin's shoulder, and loudly say, "Annie, Annie, are you okay?" But when declaring a person dead, how do you introduce yourself? Was it even necessary?

I could be in the wrong room, and if that were the case, an introduction could save some embarrassment.

I stared at the patient. His chest wasn't falling and rising. I couldn't hear him breathing.

I glanced around again, and then pushed his shoulder with my fingers. "I'm Dr. Austin," I said in a conversational tone.

He didn't respond.

I pushed harder, making his head jostle.

No response. I pulled the covers down and put my stethoscope on his chest, over his heart. There was no "lub dub" of a heart beating, no sound of air movement in the chest. I felt for pulses at the wrist, neck, and groin. Nothing.

I rubbed hard on his sternum with my knuckles. If he were alive, he'd be glad I hadn't told the nurses to zip him up in a plastic bag. If he was dead, he wouldn't feel it. But I felt bad, scrubbing my knuckles across his bony little chest.

I watched his face while I scrubbed. No expression.

I stood there, trying to find something deep or profound in the experience. But I couldn't. He was an old, dead man, and I was a young, sleepy man. I was just the guy they called in to do the paperwork.

I quietly walked from the half-dark room into the chatter and light of the nurses' station. "Who's got the guy in room seven-oh-three?" I asked the ward clerk.

"Vickie," the ward clerk called over her shoulder. "Intern's here."

A heavy young woman looked up from the chart she'd been writing on. "I got the paperwork ready for you."

"Thanks." I walked over and sat in the chair next to hers.

"Your pen have black ink?" she asked.

"Uh, yeah."

"If you use blue ink," she explained, "they send it back, 'cause it's not legal."

"Huh."

"Something about photocopying."

That didn't make sense. Blue photocopies just fine; but why argue? I clicked my pen and squiggled out a line on a piece of scrap paper. Black ink.

She nodded and slid the form over to me.

I filled in each little block, until I got to the one marked "Time of death." I looked over to Vickie. "Do I put in the time you found him, the time I got to the room, or the time right now?"

She shrugged. "Whenever you declared him."

"I didn't look at my watch."

She looked at hers. "Just put in 4:52."

The rest of the form was easy. I finished it, and slid it back to Vickie. "Anything else?" I smiled. Never hurts to be friendly.

"Nope," she said. "That's it." She smiled back at me. "Thanks for coming so quick."

"No problem," I said. "Easiest thing I've done all night."

Walking past the old man's room, I paused—should I check one last time? I didn't need to; I'd been thorough, and so had his nurse. I knew that if I went back into his room and put my stethoscope against the bony ribs of his chest, silence was all I would hear.

I stood in the darkened hallway, feeling that a fundamental insight stood outside my grasp. Something profound, about life, death, and eternity, but the only thing that came to me was a yawn.

I rode the elevator back down to my call room. Lying down, I smoothed my hair carefully behind my head and pulled the covers up to my chest, hoping to steal another hour of sleep—a down payment against the needs that the morning would bring.

VENTILATOR

Mr. Woods grinned when I walked into his room in the ICU. He raised his eyebrows and lifted his hand in a jaunty wave. His hair, usually carefully combed, was a mess over his bald spot. His nose had a subtle crook in it, just like my dad's. His black hair, thinning on the top, looked like Dad's, too.

"Good morning," I said. "How was your night?" At five forty-five, it was still dark outside, and the window looked like an obsidian mirror. The fluorescent lights of the ICU made it difficult to keep track of time. Near the end of my internship, I'd gotten used to working in the early mornings and late nights.

He jammed two thumbs in the air, nodded, and raised his eyebrows again. Maybe he'd gotten used to life on the unit as well.

"Good." I smiled back at him and nodded. I glanced at his monitor. The wave form of the silently bouncing green line was reassuringly normal; the numbers for his blood pressure, heart rate, and oxygenation were good, too. "Any problems?"

Mr. Woods shook his head, and turned the corners of his mouth down, as if to say "Piece of cake." He couldn't actually say, "Piece of cake," because several weeks previously, a surgeon had taken him to the OR, made an incision into the front of his neck, and slipped a short plastic tube into his trachea. Mr. Woods needed the tracheotomy because he'd become dependent on the ventilator to breathe for him and we couldn't wean him off of it.

"I'm glad your night was good," I said, wondering how good his night could've been, propped up in a bed in an ICU, a blue crinkly tube connecting him to a ventilator that puffed humidified air into his lungs through the tube in his neck.

Mr. Woods had been on the ventilator for several weeks because he'd suffered a respiratory arrest from COPD. Chronic obstructive pulmonary disease is almost always the result of smoking. You can think of your lungs as microscopic clusters of spherical air pockets, resembling little bunches of hollow grapes. The stems represent the tubes through which air flows to the hollowed-out little grapes, where oxygen diffuses across a thin membrane, into the surrounding network of blood-filled capillaries.

Smoking, over years, had destroyed the walls between the tiny air pockets in Mr. Woods's lungs. Instead of billions of microscopic alveoli, his lungs had become large bubblelike spaces with significantly less surface area. He had to work harder and harder, and expand his lungs further and further, just to get enough air in and out to oxygenate his blood. A few weeks before I met Mr. Woods, he'd developed a bad bronchitis which had overwhelmed his limited respiratory reserve. His gasping efforts failed to supply adequate oxygen. He'd made it to the ER in time for a doc like me to slip a tube through his mouth into his trachea and hook him up to a breathing machine. After several weeks, they'd taken the tube from his mouth and replaced it with a tracheotomy, a hole the surgeon cut in the front of his neck. Day after day I'd gone in to check on him, said, "Good morning," and watched his eyebrows go up in greeting, just the way my dad's did when he was amused. My father was a smoker, too.

If Mr. Woods had been intubated for respiratory failure secondary to something reversible, like congestive heart failure, he probably would've already been weaned off the ventilator. Congestive heart failure results in fluid building up in the lungs, prohibiting the exchange of oxygen. In those cases, you can intubate the patient, give them a diuretic to pee off the excess fluid, and then pull the tube out when the lungs clear. The machines have little dials on them, and you can incrementally dial back the amount of ventilatory support they offer. As the patient improves, you dial the ventilator back, until he can breathe on his own. But smoking had destroyed so much of Mr. Woods's lung tissue that he'd gotten stuck on the machine.

Any doc or nurse who's worked in a VA hospital can tell you about seeing a patient hunched over in a wheelchair, holding a cigarette up to the tracheotomy hole at the front of his neck, puffing away. You'd think that after smoking had damaged a patient's body to the point he'd had to have a tracheotomy, he'd quit. Of course, if it were easy to quit smoking, most people, knowing the health risks, would've already quit. But I hated the thought of my dad sticking a cigarette to a hole in the front of his neck, or ending up on a ventilator, like Mr. Woods.

The machine puffed and Mr. Woods's lungs expanded.

"Today we may try to wean you down a little further," I said. "You feel up for it?"

He scowled with mock ferocity and raised both fists, then gave me a double thumbs-up. He was ready for the fight.

"Good." I wanted to clap him on the shoulder but was afraid it would seem condescending.

"I'll check back with you later." I had three other patients to see before rounds.

He winked at me.

I winked back, and walked out of his room to the nurses' station. Mr. Woods had been the first patient assigned to me that month. He was my favorite, even though I hadn't been able to get him weaned off his ventilator. Until I did, he'd stay in the unit, and on our service. I felt pressured to keep moving my patients forward and off the service, because if I didn't, I'd have too many patients, and the other team members would have to take all the new patients. A patient you couldn't budge was called a slug.

I didn't like thinking of Mr. Woods as a slug. Slugs were people who wanted to stay in the hospital, even though they were medically well enough to go home: lonely old people whose family wouldn't take them back. Slugs were dependent, whiny, demanding people. Mr. Woods never made any demands. Of course, he couldn't talk, and didn't seem to like writing on the small dry-erase board the nurse had given him. But other intubated patients could be very demanding, snapping their fingers, scowling, and scribbling long diatribes about how miserable they were.

In the nurses' station, I opened Mr. Woods's chart and flipped through the nurses' reports. Nothing new. Each patient room had a large window looking out to the nurses' station. I looked through the slats of the Venetian blinds and watched Mr. Woods. Every time he took a breath, the machine puffed, and helped expand his lungs. He lay on the bed, his eyes closed, his face passive.

I checked on my other patients, and went downstairs to the cafeteria for breakfast before we rounded with the attending physician. The hospital gave us meal tickets for the nights we were on call. I used one to get some yogurt and an apple. I had money left over, so I got a Snickers bar and put it in the pocket of my white coat, for later. I ate quickly and went back up to the unit.

We began rounding on the patients when Dr. Solters, the ICU attending, arrived. We started with Mr. Woods.

"Any progress with the wean?" Dr. Solters asked. He was a short, wiry guy who fostered a reputation for being gruff and direct. On our first day of the ICU rotation, he'd stood in his shirt-sleeves, with his hands on his hips. "Every resident kills three patients in the process of learning to be a doctor." He shrugged. "Probably unavoidable, but don't punch all three tickets on this rotation." He grinned, glancing at each of us. "Okay?"

I tried to keep the surprise from showing on my face. Was he serious? I knew *I* hadn't killed anyone, and I hadn't heard of any avoidable deaths, except one surgery resident who'd accidentally pulled a clamp loose during surgery. The patient bled to death right there in front of them. There must've been other mistakes we'd made, but it's not like we were on the Grim Reaper's payroll.

"And I don't want anyone to die in *my* ICU without knowing about it early on. If someone's getting really sick, call me, and I'll come in and help." He paused. "If you fiddle around with them until they code, there won't be much I can do. Any questions?"

I shook my head along with the rest of the residents. He sounded cavalier, but at least he wanted to be called and would come in to help. It seemed like most of the other attendings would rather sleep through the night at home, and hear about problems the next morning.

In the pecking order of a teaching hospital, surgeons are the aggressive big dogs; then comes internal medicine, then pediatrics, then psychiatry. Within surgery, of course, cardiac surgeons lord it over general surgeons. And in medicine, interventional cardiologists, the ones who can do cardiac catheterizations, are the big dogs; then come the ICU docs, and then the general internists. Until a cardiologist or surgeon walked up, Dr. Solters was a pretty cocky guy.

ER docs are kind of off to the side. We're good at working in chaos and under tight time constraints. A good ER doc can keep a lot going at the same time. Most docs in other specialties understand this, or at least pretend to, and they give us a little credit for what we do. Can a cardiologist do a better job with a heart attack than an ER doc? I hope so; otherwise, they wasted three years after residency, getting their subspecialty training. But can they do the first ten minutes as well as an ER doc? Some of them can, some of them can't. It's hard to stay calm and bring order to the initial chaos. Paramedics are telling you what the patient looked like when they first arrived, nurses are busy popping off the paramedics' monitor leads and snapping ours in place, the aluminum wrench clanks against the green oxygen bottle, people call out they need this or that. The other specialists may know more about any given disease than we do, but most of them couldn't handle the chaos as well. So, although we're not the big dogs, most ER docs have sufficient ego to walk out into the ER and pick up a chart and go see the patient, no matter what the problem is.

"The wean has been slow," I said to Dr. Solters, glancing in through the slats of the Venetian blinds on Mr. Woods's window.

Mr. Woods smiled and waved.

I smiled back, and nodded, but was too embarrassed to wave because the whole team was watching. "As soon as we get close to a wean, he tires out."

"Smoker." Dr. Solters shrugged. "Any questions, concerns?"

"Not really," I said. "Guess I'll just keep dialing him back in really small increments."

Dr. Solters nodded, and led our small herd of white coats to the patient next door. As the other resident discussed his new patient, I wrote an order in Mr. Woods's chart to dial back on his ventilator settings. I handed the chart to Hannah, his nurse. Some of the ICU nurses wore scrubs with patterns—little frogs with stethoscopes, Teddy bears in nurses' uniforms. Hannah wore unisex green scrub tops tucked into the waist of unisex bottoms. A small golden cross glowed against the dark skin at the notch at the base of her throat. Her hair was a short, tight afro.

"Okay." Hannah took the chart and placed it on the small desk outside Mr. Woods's room. I couldn't tell if she expected the wean to work. She'd been an ICU nurse for several years, and I trusted her judgment, but the team had moved on, and I didn't have time to ask her.

Later that morning, Hannah asked me to come check Mr. Woods. "He's not going to fly." She looked from the ventilator to Mr. Woods's face.

It must have been a nightmare for Mr. Woods, unable to get off the machine that kept him alive but also kept him tethered to the same bed, in the same room, week after week. When I was a kid, I had asthma, and I remember the frantic feeling that I was being held underwater, clawing my way up toward the air. I'd sit in bed, leaning forward, focusing every ounce of my energy on getting one more breath in, one more breath out, one more breath in, one more breath out. Mom would rub Vicks VapoRub on my chest and put a dab under my nose. The eucalyptus made the inside of my nose sting, but other than that, didn't do much. But it was the only thing medicine had to offer in the 1960s, short of a trip to the ER for a shot of epinephrine. She used what she had.

Mr. Woods sat straight up in bed, hunching his shoulders with each breath, trying to pull more air in through the skinny tube in his neck. He pointed to his dry-erase board.

Hannah handed him the board and a marker.

In wavering letters, he wrote: "More air." His hands trembled as he recapped the marker.

"I can tell you're short of breath," I said.

He bobbed his head in an impatient nod. *No shit.*

"If we can just tough it out a little longer," I said, "we'll probably be able to get you off this forever."

He raised his eyebrows, as if suspending judgment. He carefully uncapped the marker. "OK," he wrote in wavy letters. He closed his eyes.

Thirty minutes later, the alarms on the ventilator started dinging.

Hannah came and got me.

Mr. Woods sat in bed with his eyes closed. The muscles in his neck stood out with the effort of each breath.

Mr. Woods's efforts made my shoulders and neck muscles feel tight, and made me want to take a full, deep breath.

"He's tiring out," I said to Hannah. I took a long, deep, silent breath.

She nodded.

The decision to keep trying or give up was partially dependent on personalities. Mr. Woods didn't seem like a quitter. If he could make it, he would. But it was hard to tell. Hannah had seen more

COPD patients weaned from ventilators than I had, which wasn't hard, since this was my first. But she cared about Mr. Woods, and seemed competent. I was grateful for her help.

"Mr. Woods," I said, "it looks like we may need to go back up on your vent settings."

He nodded in defeated acquiescence. He didn't look at me.

"Don't worry," I said. "We'll try again."

Mr. Woods closed his eyes.

We turned the vent settings back up, and Mr. Woods's chest expanded fully. Poor guy. On one hand, we had a treatment that was brutally effective in helping him breathe, but on the other, we couldn't get him off of it.

My dad smoked. He didn't have any hobbies, other than books and his pipe collection. I wasn't allowed to touch his meerschaum pipe, because it would break if I dropped it. Dad explained how the bowl would turn to a deep reddish-brown with use. I kept checking to see if it had changed, but week after week it was that same ivory color. Turns out he was talking about years of use.

I never liked cigarette smoke. It made me cough and wheeze, and it smelled bad. But who can resist the deep, complex aromas of a pipe? When I put my nose to the empty bowl of one of Dad's pipes, it stank. But when he'd gently tamp the tobacco, and suck the fire from a match into the pipe, the whole room became rich with its aroma. In the years before my parents' divorce, Dad would sit in his chair for hours, reading and smoking pipes or cigarettes.

Everyone knows smoking isn't good for you, but in my second year of medical school, I found out that sure enough, smoking kills people. We had a lecture on smoking cessation, in which we were taught new techniques, and learned the results of recent research. I called Dad. "I had a lecture today about smoking."

The line was silent. "Paul," Dad finally said, "I've tried to quit. You don't know how many times."

"I know," I said. "But every time you quit, you increase the odds that the next time will be successful." I was proud I could tell my father about the latest research.

"I appreciate your concern," Dad said, "but this isn't something I want to talk about."

Is there anything worse than a religious nut who won't leave you alone, keeps yammering at you about whether you're really, really saved? That's how I must've seemed to Dad, with my repeated attempts to reopen the discussion about smoking.

He finally told me there was no point in bringing it up again. I knew I was in an absurd position. Go off to medical school, get a couple of lectures about smoking cessation, and try to change the world. Bottom line, he was the dad, I was the son.

On my last day on the intensive care unit, I said good-bye to each of my patients. I went to see Mr. Woods last. I didn't look forward to seeing him, because I felt like I'd failed him.

"It was good to know you," I said, shaking his hand.

His grip was stronger than I'd anticipated. He pointed to his chest, then to me, nodding.

"Sorry we couldn't get you off that thing," I said, pointing to the square machine beside his bed.

He glanced over at the ventilator as if it were a cranky family member. He looked me in the eyes and shrugged. I couldn't assign an emotion to his expression. Defeat? Acceptance? I didn't know.

"Better go," I said, pointing to the door.

He raised his hand, palm up, and smiled. The ventilator chugged another breath into him.

I didn't tell my dad I had a recurring nightmare that month, in which he was the intubated ICU patient hooked up to a ventilator. In my dream, I walked into my father's room and stood at the foot of his bed. The windows were black with night. Monitors and technology loomed over him, their faint green glow giving the only light to the room. He couldn't speak, and his eyes were all he could move. His eyes followed me. They looked scared, and were trying to tell me something. In my dream I turned toward the gauges and twisted the dials, relieved to be too busy to let my eyes rest on my silently frantic father.

AMONG SAVAGES

Depending on the specialty I was rotating through, I spent every third night, sometimes every other, in the hospital, on call. Those nights pulled me away from my family, but I was getting to do things that other people only watch on TV. I delivered babies, treated septic shock, and pulled dislocated shoulders back into place—I was acquiring the skills I'd be using for the rest of my career. And although it was a stressful period, I knew it would be temporary: once I finished the three years of residency training, our growing young family would be happier. We were already doing okay—John, our newborn, had arrived without any health problems, and we were able to afford for Sally to stay home with the children, something she'd always wanted to do. All we had to do was stick it out until I finished residency training.

Occasionally I'd remember Kyle, the intern I'd met when I was a nursing assistant. I hoped to acquire his sheen of competence without taking on his apparent indifference to the suffering he saw. On most rotations, I could steal a couple of hours of sleep each night, which made it easier to care about patients, or at least fake it. But on the trauma service, the relentless grind eventually peeled away my defenses, and showed me a part of myself I would have liked to deny.

One Saturday night, Fast Eddie, the chief resident, sent Jonsie McClendon and me down to the ER to check out a drunk who'd flipped his car. The paramedics had bandaged his scalp laceration, put him in a neck collar, and strapped him to a spine board before bringing him in.

The ER had asked for a trauma consult because the guy's mental status was hard to evaluate: he could just be a drunk, or he could have a closed head injury. In a car crash, the brain can get bounced around inside the skull, shearing connections. And if a vein or an artery gets torn, a blood clot grows and grows, compressing the brain until it no longer functions.

Jonsie and I walked down to begin the process of evaluating him for admission. We knew that if the guy was severely injured, the ER would have called a "trauma code," and the whole team would've rushed down to take the guy immediately to the operating room. When they called for a routine consult, the injuries were usually minor. In those cases, we usually got a bunch of CT scans, and admitted the patient overnight, just to make sure we had not missed anything.

We went to the dry-erase board in the center of the ER and found our guy's room number. Sighing, Jonsie grabbed a packet of admission paperwork and handed it to me. When we walked into the trauma bay, the ER resident gave us a quick verbal report, then ducked out of the room. The drunk guy was snoring loudly, filling the room with the smell of beer and vomit. Blood had splashed down the guy's face and onto his flannel shirt. Thick strings of partly digested food and saliva had soaked into his beard. He was a large man, his shoulders extending far past the plywood board the paramedics had strapped him to.

"Sir," Jonsie said in a loud voice, pulling on a pair of latex exam gloves he'd gotten from the box on the counter, between the contaminated needles box and IV supply box. He prodded the man's shoulder. "Are you okay?"

The guy mumbled something, and pushed Jonsie's hand away.

"He's drunk." Jonsie wiped his gloved hand on the sheet. "Ought to chew his food better, too."

"Gonna scan his head?" I started writing routine admission orders.

"Well, yeah." Jonsie snorted. "But we both know it's going to be normal."

We did a quick physical exam, looked at the X-rays the ER had made, and put in an order for a head CT. When the scan tech called and said they'd do our patient, we pushed the gurney downstairs. Even with the routine cases, Jonsie and I didn't like to wait for transporters—the sooner we got this guy tucked in, the sooner we could get back to our other work.

Down in the CT suite, we helped the tech slide our guy over to the scanner's table. Jonsie and I sat in the chilly outer area, finishing our chartwork at a desk that allowed us to observe our patient through a small glass window.

The table slowly glided into the large, open ring of the scanner. Just as his head slid in, the man woke up, started screaming, and tore off the collar the paramedics had placed around his neck. Big guy.

Jonsie yelled to the CT tech, "Call the ER, get someone to come tube this guy!" We scrambled in to hold the man down, keeping him on the scanner table until someone could come down, sedate, and intubate him before he hurt himself.

It was slippery work because he was sweaty, strong, and determined, but we kept him pinned to the table.

Years ago, if a trauma patient was too drunk to cooperate, he was left in a corner to "sleep it off" until he was sober enough to cooperate with his evaluation. Some of these patients had brain hemorrhages that were masked by the intoxication. The right way to evaluate a combative major trauma patient is to give him Vecuronium, a medication that will pharmacologically paralyze him. It's a derivative of curare, the stuff South American native people put on the tips of blowdarts to paralyze their prey. You inject the medicine, and the patient loses all motor strength. Of course when you do this, the patient can no longer breathe, so you have to insert a tube into his trachea to breathe for him.

One of my attendings from the ER came in, paralyzed the guy, and intubated him right on the scanner table.

Jonsie and I relaxed our grips as the guy went flaccid. I looked at my hands, smeared with blood and vomit because I hadn't had time to put on gloves. Jonsie looked at his, which were smeared red, too. He shook his head.

We went to wash our hands. "He'd better fucking hope he doesn't have AIDS," Jonsie said as he scrubbed. He rinsed his hands, and scrubbed again.

We both knew that the trauma attendings and Fast Eddie were going to give us a hard time about a crash tube, down in the CT scanner. "Control," they were going to say. "You had no control of the patient, his airway, or the situation." They'd cross their arms and shake their heads, as if hoping we'd learned our lesson. As soon as the attending left, Fast Eddie would say, "You get down to Scan Land with a patient without securing an airway, you're fucked."

When we got back to the scanner from washing our hands, the ER attending physician left. The drunk guy's head CT was normal. He was just drunk.

Jonsie leaned over the guy's face, immobile because he was still paralyzed from the medication. "You couldn't be a *happy* drunk, could you?" Jonsie yelled, bits of spit flicking out onto the guy's face. "Nooooooo. You had to be an *asshole.*" His voice scaled upward and the veins on the side of his neck popped out. "Now you're fucking *paralyzed.*"

I understood Jonsie's frustration. And I knew the drunk probably wouldn't remember Jonsie yelling at him in the morning. But damn—I knew I'd never yell at a patient like that. Still, I envied Jonsie's catharsis.

Jonsie, the CT technician, and I put on gloves and pulled the drunk over to our ER stretcher. Jonsie and I wheeled the guy up to the trauma intensive care unit, where we moved him onto a bed.

Many of our patients are intoxicated when they come in. Sometimes, a sober guy will show up. A tree trimmer who's fallen thirty feet, or a sober driver who's wrecked his car. They are easier to take care of, because they know they've been injured and want to do anything they can to help us take care of them. Even some of the patients who are intoxicated are easy to work with. "Whatever," they'll say, with a benign wave of the hand. But others will argue with the cops, with the nurses, with the docs, anyone who has to talk to them. And it gets tiresome. Real, real tiresome. Especially for the residents who plan to go into general surgery, or plastics, where they won't have to interact with drunks. As an ER resident, I knew drunks would be a significant part of my working life, so I wanted to get good at dealing with them. I thought it was possible. I couldn't know that later in my trauma rotation, a drunk would cause me serious problems.

During my first month on the trauma service I went with Jim Spangler, one of the other surgery residents, to babysit a drunk in the ER. Three thirty in the morning, on our tenth admission. We'd been up all night. I felt a buzzing need to sleep.

Jim and I walked into the X-ray room. Melinda, an ER intern I didn't know that well, leaned against the wall next to the patient's gurney. "Lay flat, sir," she said in a bored monotone. "Don't lift your head, sir. Your neck might be broken."

The drunk struggled to lift his head. "My neck isn't broke," he slurred.

The intern gently pressed down on his forehead. "You're intoxicated, sir," Melinda said. "You could have a fracture and not know it." She was, of course, right. Intoxication is one of the documented risk factors for having an undiagnosed cervical spine fracture.

"I'm not that fucking drunk," he said, lifting his head again.

When Melinda saw us, she stripped off her latex gloves. She motioned to the guy with her head. "Unrestrained driver, not ejected, steering wheel bent, windshield starred. Stable vital signs. He's been like this since he got here." She paused, to see if we had any questions.

We didn't. I was impressed that she had the rap down so tight within the first months of internship. Of course, she'd already had lots of practice.

She left.

The drunk raised his head and tried to look at us, but his collar limited his motion. "Put your head down, sir," Jim said, as he leafed through the paperwork on the clipboard. I started writing his admission orders.

The drunk continued to try to look at us.

"Put your head down, sir," Jim repeated, a sharper edge to his voice.

"My neck isn't broke," the drunk said again.

"Put your head *down*, sir."

"Fuck you." The drunk tried to spit at us.

Jim grabbed the guy's hair and snapped his head back onto the plywood backboard, his face inches from the drunk's. "Listen, dickhead. You fuck yourself up on my watch, and *my* ass is in trouble." He thumped the guy's head against the board again. "Got that?"

The drunk nodded his head, in the small arc the collar permitted.

"Stop moving your fucking head." Jim went back to the chartwork.

I wished there was a way I could've warned the man: "Buddy, it's way past midnight and you've fallen among savages. Do what we say, you won't get hurt." Of course, I'd already discovered the futility of reasoning or pleading with drunks. Jim's method had the advantage of simplicity, clarity, and honesty. It just wouldn't sound good to anyone who hadn't been in our position. "Sir," I said, "wiggle your toes and fingers."

He did.

The guy had on a neck collar, and I knew Jim thumping the

guy's head against the board wasn't that likely to exacerbate whatever injury he might have, but I wanted to establish that he was still in as good a shape as when we'd taken over.

"He's fine," Jim said. "Fucking indestructible."

Some drunks are like Otis, the bumbling, amiable guy on *The Andy Griffith Show*. Others are like the ones you remember from college, playing drinking games—laughing, carefree souls. And some can be snappy, sharp-tongued, saying outrageous things that challenge the pomposity of docs and nurses. By and large, the worst they may do would be to try to flirt with the nurses, or grab at a nurse's ass as she walks by.

But other drunks, the ones who've gotten in fights or wrecks trying to outrun the cops, are combative, angry, dangerous people. And we all know that the same guy who spits at you through bloody lips and calls you motherfucker will be sober when he sues you if there's a bad outcome in his care. In court, his face will be freshly shaved, his hair carefully combed. He'll be contrite for having been intoxicated. His lawyer will be baffled by the way doctors let him injure himself while he was incapacitated.

To let hostility show is a failure. A failure of boundaries, a failure of self-control. If you counted on human compassion to keep you from smacking one of these guys, you'd be in trouble by the third day on the job. And if you let them get to you to the point where it shows, you have no business being an ER doc.

On one level, taking care of drunk patients became just another aspect of the trauma service I had to get used to—part of the price I had to pay to get the training I needed. Like the cold, drab weather in Pittsburgh, complaining about it wouldn't change a thing, so I tried not to talk about it too much at home.

I had so little time off, I hated to waste it thinking about the hospital.

Sally and I had now been married six years. She had worked part time, as a nurse, in a different hospital, until John, our second child, was born. We didn't have a cradle when John arrived, so we pulled a drawer from a maple dresser, padded it, and placed it next to our bed. Sally could lean over, pick him up, nurse him, and put him back in his drawer without getting up.

Sarah, four years old, went to a day care with special education teachers and occupational therapists. She'd been labeled as "high functioning," and when they tested her IQ, it was only a few points away from low-normal.

Sally and I, like all couples, had things we had to deal with: Sarah's Down syndrome, a new infant, moving to a new city, the chronic exhaustion of residency training.

So, if I had a weekend when I wasn't on call, I didn't want to think or talk about work. I'd rather build a sandbox in the backyard for Sarah, or take a walk with Sally, pushing Sarah in the stroller or carrying John in one of those baby backpacks, up and down the hills of the working-class Pittsburgh neighborhood in which we lived.

In the second month on the trauma service, I was at home, eating supper with Sally and Sarah. John was upstairs, sleeping in his drawer. The phone rang—my dad. When they'd divorced years earlier, Dad had remarried; Mom hadn't. As one would expect, they'd both wanted me to take their side. Both had told me things about their relationship I didn't want to know, and both had leaned on me too frequently. I'd finally gotten a cushion of time and distance between me and my parents' divorce, but I still felt a wariness when either one called.

"Paul," he said, his voice shaking, "I've got lung cancer." He paused, and continued, "I'm scheduled to have it taken out in two days."

"Oh, Dad." Fucking *lung cancer*? I felt myself retreat from the news.

"I feel guilty," he said, "for calling you like this."

"Guilty?" I asked. *For having lung cancer?*

"It's my own fault." He coughed. "The smoking all these years." He coughed again and cleared his throat. "I feel like I brought this on myself." His voice rasped. I couldn't tell if something was hung in his throat, or if it was from the emotional pressure of what he was trying to say. "So I'm sorry."

"Don't worry about any of that," I said. "The only thing that matters is you getting well." I stared down at the black-and-red-square pattern of the linoleum in our kitchen.

The line was silent. I looked up at Sally, who quietly put her fork down on her plate. Sarah stared at me as she slowly gnawed on the string bean she clutched in her fist.

"So." Dad cleared his throat. "I'm going to have it removed in a couple of days."

"Where?"

"At the hospital here."

"Let me talk to someone at UNC." My hometown hospital was reputable, but I wanted Dad to have the best.

"No," Dad said. "I trust the surgeon here. You'd like him. A real straight shooter."

"Chapel Hill's only a couple of hours away."

"Paul, the decision's been made."

"Okay. I'll come down tomorrow," I said, wondering how I'd work it out with the trauma team.

"You don't have to do that," he said. "The surgeon said it should be quick and simple."

Quick and simple—lung cancer? "Dad, I want to be there. I'll call tomorrow." We hung up.

"Is he okay?" Sally asked. She reached for my hand.

"Has a lung mass." I took Sally's hand, our fingers interlaced. "Local surgeon's going to resect it in two days."

"Are you going down?"

"I'll try to." I hoped Fast Eddie would let me go. I didn't want to take it up the chain of command, but if I had to, I would.

There's a macho culture in surgery, and trauma surgery offers its ultimate manifestation. It's like the boys' locker room in junior high. Lots of bullying and joking. The overriding culture is: "Don't complain, don't explain." I'd first experienced such a culture in Catholic high school. I'd grown up Quaker and had been in public school all through elementary and junior high school, but when I was in tenth grade, my parents put me in Bishop McGuinness Memorial High School. I'd never heard a Hail Mary or seen a nun, except on TV. I learned quickly that the most efficient way to navigate a problem with a nun was to say, "Yes, Sister," "No, Sister," or, "It won't happen again, Sister." Same thing in the fire department. If a piece of equipment was missing or broken or misplaced, the only sane response a firefighter could give was, "No excuse, sir. It won't happen again." I was luckier than some of my fellow residents who'd been the best and the brightest all the way through school. They seemed to think an attending surgeon would give a rat's ass about why they'd made a mistake, or how it really wasn't their fault.

On the trauma service, I felt like I was finally learning how to get along with surgeons. It isn't an easy thing to do. There's a whole mystique, a whole catechism you must learn, to go into an operating room. It involves sterility and etiquette. Both aspects of the endeavor have value. Sterility must be scrupulously maintained. And if a medical student is in the way, a surgeon could make a mistake. A scrub nurse teaches the medical students how to scrub in. You wash your hands carefully, scrubbing each finger ten strokes on the front, back, and each side. Then you scrub the palm ten times, then the back ten times, then the forearm ten times. The water cuts on and off with foot pedals. When you're done washing and rinsing, you hold your forearms up in the air, like a supplicant, so the water drips down from your fingers, to your elbow, then to the floor. If you held your hands down, dirty water from your elbow would sluice down over your clean hands.

I enjoyed the ritual, the calming time of scrubbing, getting fastidiously clean. As you back into the OR, butt-first to open the door, a scrub nurse hands you a sterile towel that you use to dry off. Hands first, then wrists, then forearms, always going from sterile to non-sterile. Then you toss the towel into a hamper, and the scrub nurse helps you into a sterile gown. I felt like a prince, or a rich man having help from a tailor, as I reached in with my left arm then my right, twirling around, so the scrub nurse could sterilely hand me the tie at my waist.

Then the nurse holds out a sterile glove and you push your hand down into it, trying not to get two fingers into one slot. You feel a lot like a clumsy kid whose mom's helping you get ready to go outside in the snow. If your fingers get crossed up, you can undo them when you get your other glove on. Then you stand, waiting to be motioned toward the patient. Like getting on a boat, you wait for permission. You do not speak. You put both hands on the sterile patient and leave them there, to make sure you don't let them stray to a non-sterile place.

I enjoyed the OR. If it was an abdominal case, the surgeon often needed someone to hold a retractor, the stainless steel curved strap the surgeon would use to pull the intestines—a glistening, pale blue-white mass of squishiness—out of the way. And you'd hold the retractor, and get to watch, or daydream.

We also scrubbed in on cardiac cases. A bypass graft is a big operation that involves splitting the sternum in half and opening the chest like a clamshell. On the case I scrubbed in on, a physician's assistant harvested vein from the patient's leg for the surgeon to use when he made the bypass around the clogged portion of the coronary artery. I was allowed to sew up the leg, a low-skill endeavor. When I was done, I could watch the surgeon operate on the naked human heart.

Once, while scrubbed in on a coronary artery bypass surgery, the attending accidentally smacked me on the head with an elbow.

"Sleeve," he then called out, turning from the table.

My head, non-sterile, had contaminated the sleeve of his gown. "Sorry, sir," I said.

"It's okay," he said, although he'd been the one to elbow me.

An OR nurse hustled over with a sterile paper sleeve with elastic at both ends. She held one end open for him.

"Just don't let it happen again," he said, as he plunged his hand down into the paper tube. He turned back to the patient's chest and held out his hand. "Scalpel."

I moved away.

He didn't notice me for the rest of the surgery. That suited me fine. On one level, he seemed like an asshole. On the other, if I had my hands in someone's chest, I wouldn't want a medical student crowding me. Of course, I think I'd ask them to give me a little room, rather than just smack them with an elbow.

Most of the surgery attendings and residents were good guys—and they were guys. There was only one woman in the general surgery program when I was there, and she bailed out. Surgeons reminded me of jocks—optimistic, not very introspective, quintessentially American: "Let's fix it." I liked that attitude, but their training didn't seem to allow for much human weakness. And family leave was just as weak as maternity leave, so I was afraid they'd give me a lot of shit about wanting to get off work.

The next morning, I told Fast Eddie I needed to leave that night. "My dad's going in for a partial pneumonectomy tomorrow," I said. "I'd like to be there."

He looked up from the chart he was working on. "Where's he getting it done?"

"My hometown hospital."

"Ouch," he said, wincing. "Can't you get him up here? Stone would do him." Dr. Stone was one of the cardiothoracic surgeons who was regionally famous. Did experimental heart surgery. They'd named a wing of the hospital after him.

"Dad likes the guy down there."

"When is it?"

"Tomorrow," I said. "I'd like to leave tonight."

"You on call?"

"I am tomorrow night."

Eddie winced again, then said, "Don't worry. Jonsie can cover for you."

"Thanks."

"But you can tell him."

"Okay." I went to the nurses' station, called home, and asked Sally to get me a plane ticket for that night. After I'd graduated from medical school, our mailbox had been flooded with offers for credit cards and unsecured loans, so I wasn't worried about how I would pay for the plane fare.

I paged Jonsie, and when he called back, told him about my dad. He said he'd take my call for me. If you worked hard and didn't complain, even if you were an ER resident rotating through trauma surgery, the team would take care of you. I thanked him and promised to pay him back.

That afternoon, Sally paged me. My flight was at seven o'clock. If I left the hospital at five thirty, I'd get home by six, grab a suitcase, leave, and get to the airport by six thirty. I could shower at Dad's house. If I could leave the hospital half an hour earlier, which was early for the trauma service, I'd have a little more leeway. I asked Eddie if I could get out by five.

"What?" He frowned, his eyes screwed up into a squint.

"I'd like to get out a little early. I gotta be at the airport by six thirty."

"Airport?" He looked over at me. "Oh yeah, your dad." He nodded, and slapped me on the shoulder. "Don't worry," he said. "We'll get you out."

At 4:30 P.M., I got a page, and returned it. "Paul," Eddie said. "Go down to the ER, babysit some drunk that just came in. Unrestrained driver, ejected, never hypotensive. I know you gotta catch a plane, I'll get Jonsie to relieve you in plenty of time." He hung up before I could say anything. Must've had a problem upstairs.

I got on the elevator and jabbed the first-floor button. Some asshole had wrecked his car, and was going to moan and bitch. He'd pull at the chin of his cervical collar, and wiggle his toes. "See? I don't need no fucking X-rays." *Yeah, yeah, yeah. But when you move your neck and paralyze yourself from the shoulders down, in a year or two you'll get all dressed up in a nice dark suit and sit in a wheelchair in the front of the courtroom, staring straight at me.*

I walked into the ER. "Where's the trauma?" I asked one of my classmates.

"X-ray," she replied. "You okay?"

No. I am not okay. I'm babysitting some drunk instead of going to see my dad. I kept on walking without replying.

In the X-ray room a guy was lying on a plywood backboard, and the X-ray technician was taping a film cassette beside his neck.

"Fuck you people," the drunk shouted. "I told you, I don't need no X-rays." He fumbled with the Velcro tabs securing his neck collar. "Get me off this fucking board!" He tried to sit up.

I rushed to the stretcher, jammed my face into his, and shouted, "Shut up!"

He blinked as my spit hit his eyes.

"My name is Dr. Austin, A-U-S-T-I-N, and you're going to *shut* up and *lay* down." I ached to vent more of my pent-up anger but knew that I couldn't. I was afraid that my father's cancer could kill him, I was mad that I'd been delayed in getting to the airport, and furious that I had to babysit yet another drunk in the ER. My rage and restraint were perfectly balanced—but if the guy spit on me, or cursed me, I'd bust his face.

That must've registered, because he put his head down quietly.

His breath had the sweetly rotten smell of alcohol. I straightened, and took a deep breath. The two X-ray technicians and the nurse stared at me, their mouths open.

"What?" I demanded, looking around the room.

They glanced at each other, then back at me again.

"Well," I asked, "you-all gonna make the X-rays, or not?"

The X-ray techs started moving again, talking quietly among themselves while adjusting the dials on their machines.

While one X-ray tech put the film in the processor, the nurse told the patient, "Sir, I'm going to put in a Foley catheter."

"What?" he asked, trying to lift his head off the stretcher.

I rushed over and put my face into his again. "All you're going to do is shut up and hold still."

He let his head fall back on the board.

As the nurse pushed the thin rubber tube up into the guy's penis, he hummed loudly.

I let him hum.

The X-ray techs took the last film, and the nurse and I wheeled the drunk back to his bay in the ER.

Leaning over a stainless steel stand, I started writing out the history and physical. I wanted to stay busy, so I wouldn't worry about missing my plane. Jonsie hurried in. "Sorry I'm late," he said. "Had a little problem upstairs."

"It's okay," I said, as I handed him the paperwork. "I got the H and P done, but haven't finished the orders." I turned to go, then stopped. "Thanks, Jonsie," I said. "I owe you one."

"It's your dad," he said, looking up from the chart. "Forget this fucking place."

"Thanks." I rode the elevator to the lower level of the hospital. The doors slid open. I walked down the underground hallway toward the parking deck. I was glad no one was there, because I felt tears coming and wasn't sure I could control them. Jonsie's words, "It's your dad. Forget this fucking place," seemed like the wisest, kindest words I'd ever heard, and they threatened to open up feelings that I feared would overwhelm me. At the end of the hallway, I took a deep breath and let it out as I waited for the elevator. The doors slid open, and I rode to the third level, where I'd parked that morning, and stepped out into the pale gray evening.

I glanced at my watch: 6:05. We lived about twelve minutes from the hospital and twenty minutes from the airport, so if I skipped a shower, I'd make my flight in time.

At home, I stripped off my scrubs: 6:20. I jumped into a pair of jeans and a T-shirt. I stuffed some clothes into a suitcase, kissed Sally, and drove to the airport, drumming the steering wheel with my fingers. I parked in the expensive lot, right next to the terminal, and jogged to the check-in counter. I glanced at my watch: 6:45.

"You'll have to hurry, sir," the lady said, as she hefted my suitcase onto the conveyor belt behind her counter. "They're boarding now. Gate Twenty-Two."

I ran.

The flight attendants were checking the overhead compartments as I slipped into my seat and buckled the belt. I took slow, deep breaths and closed my eyes. I didn't want to talk to the person sitting next to me, and I didn't want to read the magazine in the pouch in front of me. I just wanted to sit, and feel the jet accelerate forward and upward, toward my father.

FACE-TO-FACE

"YOU'LL like Dr. Gardner," Dad said. I was sitting in the backseat, and Dad looked at me in the rearview mirror, then back to the road exiting the airport. "He's straightforward. Says the mass is on the outer surface of the lung, and shouldn't be too hard to get out."

"That's good," I said. I still thought he should have it done in Chapel Hill.

When Dad and Judie, his wife, picked me up from the airport, he looked frail and old. His hug was tentative, and my return hug was careful. I'd told him on the phone that I would get a cab, but he wanted to pick me up.

"Dr. Gardner's the best surgeon in town," Judie added.

"Good," I said, as I glanced out the car window. *Small pond, big fish*. The hospital where I was in training kept three helicopters in the air, flying in patients whose local facilities had failed to provide enough expertise. The thought of Dad's ribs being splayed open in a small-town hospital worried me.

"You didn't have to come down for this, Paul," Dad said, looking back at me again. "But I'm glad you did."

When we got to Dad and Judie's house, we sat in their den,

talking about books and the public library he directed. Judie listened as she knitted. At ten o'clock, Dad looked at his watch. "I'd better get some sleep," he said. "Big day tomorrow."

I didn't want to think about him lying on his side, and the surgeon running a scalpel into his chest. "You'll do fine." I'd come down with a notion of helping somehow, but there wasn't really much for me to do. The only medical advice I was competent to offer was to go to a major medical center for the surgery. Dad had already rejected that. But maybe my presence as his son had value.

The next day, at the hospital, Judie went with Dad through all the pre-op stuff, while I sat in the waiting room, flipping through magazines. When I first started working in the ER as a nursing assistant, I'd felt uncomfortable walking through the hospital. The corridors had seemed as hushed as a church or a funeral parlor, and the cheerful efficiency of the nurses had seemed somehow incongruous. But after spending a couple of years there, I'd begun to feel at home.

As a resident, I sometimes wondered what it was like for the people in the waiting rooms. Fear must be a part of it, but there was also an excitement, a break in the routine. A brush against death that galvanized your attention, but that hopefully wouldn't leave anyone permanently scarred. I got up, used the bathroom, and got another cup of coffee. I waited. If I'd been a thoracic surgeon, I'd probably be feeling torn, wanting to *do* something. But I was just a resident in emergency medicine, and there wasn't anything for me to do: I was relieved to know someone else was responsible, even if it was a local guy.

A lady with white hair and a pink volunteer jacket carefully wrote the name of each visitor in a log book. She looked just like the volunteers back in Pittsburgh. The overhead pager sounded southern, but otherwise could be paging doctors at the hospital where I was training. The sights and sounds were familiar from working in the hospital, but I wasn't a young doctor—I was just another nervous family member. The room was warm, and the months of sleep deprivation were catching up to me. I felt my head bob.

"Dr. Austin?" I heard a loud, hearty voice.

"Yes!" I startled awake and stood.

"Barry Gardner," a tall man said. "I'll be operating on your father." His smile appeared confident, genuine. The backs of his hands carried traces of the white talcum powder that dusts the insides of surgical gloves. "Good to meet you." His handshake was brisk, firm.

"Come on," he said, turning. "You can keep him company in pre-op." He walked fast, and I trotted to catch up. "Neal says you're in residency training for ER," he said, over his shoulder.

"Yes," I said, hustling to keep up.

"Great specialty," he said. "When you're off, you're really off." He stopped and looked over at me. "Want to scrub in on your father's surgery?"

"Uhh, thanks," I said. "But I can wait with Judie."

"Okay," he said, turning to walk again. "Should be pretty simple. CT shows it's close to the surface."

I hoped he didn't feel rebuffed, but I really didn't want to watch Dad with an endotracheal tube snaking out of his mouth, or see his ribs spread open like a largemouth bass.

In the pre-op area, Dad was lying on a stretcher. A short woman in green scrubs was keeping him and Judie company.

"Georgianna," Dr. Gardner said, "my physician's assistant." He gestured toward me. "Neal's son. He's in residency for ER."

Georgianna and I shook hands. "Your father's told me all about you," she said, smiling. "There's coffee in the doctors' lounge if you'd like a cup."

"Thanks," I said, "but I'm fine." I wondered if Dad and Judie were glad I was in the same club as Dr. Gardner, or wished he would focus more on Dad's lung mass and less on his son's future profession. Dr. Gardner seemed capable. Enthusiastic, straightforward, as Dad had said. Maybe lung masses were so routine he made small talk about other stuff, to keep it interesting.

"Well," Dr. Gardner said. "Better go get scrubbed." He sounded as if he couldn't wait to get started. He turned to walk through the pair of double doors marked NO ADMITTANCE.

Georgianna smiled at us. "We'll take good care of you," she said to Dad. Turning to me, she said, "I just love the chest cases."

"Oh?" I said. "What other cases do you-all do?"

"Everything. Hernias, gallbladders, appendices. I like the chest cases best."

"Oh." I nodded. *Great, my dad's going to have his chest opened by a guy who usually mucks around with gallbladders.*

"Well," she said, "I guess I better go scrub in, too." She hurried after Dr. Gardner.

Did Dad know a general surgeon was opening up his chest? I imagined a series of surgical complications. The surgeon's hands would be buried in Dad's chest as a thin jet of arterial blood spurted out and splashed his face. "These guys can get tricky," he'd say to Georgianna, who'd wipe the blood from his eyes. Dr. Gardner would fumble around in the deep recesses of Dad's chest, as blood cascaded around his hands, then say, "Can we get one of the thoracic guys in here to help? This pulmonary artery just keeps slipping through my clamp." A scrub nurse would hurry out of the room to go get help. The anesthesiologist would mutter something about the dropping blood pressure, Dr. Gardner would tersely reply, and Georgianna would stand quietly with her hands resting on Dad's chest . . .

A few minutes later, a nurse in green scrubs walked up. "Ready?" she asked Dad.

"You bet."

Judie patted his shoulder, and the nurse wheeled my dad through the double doors. Judie and I walked to the cafeteria for coffee and went back to the waiting room. Judie pulled a ball of green yarn and a pair of knitting needles from her pocketbook. I liked her practical approach to life, and wished my parents had let go of the hostility that kept churning up around their divorce. I couldn't shake the feeling that I was betraying Mom by spending time with Dad. Even after all those years, the possibility of liking my dad's wife felt like a renunciation of my mother. But sitting in the vinyl chair of a waiting room as a hometown doctor slipped a scalpel between my father's ribs, the settling dust of my family's collapse seemed less important. And my parents' failed marriage was beyond my control, just like the small clump of cancerous cells growing in my father's lung. All I could do was sit and wait.

Dad would be okay. His primary doctor wouldn't send him to someone who wasn't competent. And an attending doctor who's been doing it for years would do a better job than an intern in some academic center, for whom it would be the first or second time he'd done the operation. A general surgeon working carefully also would do a better job than a thoracic specialist, who might get cocky because the case was so routine. I shifted in my chair. Dr. Gardner wouldn't have invited me to scrub in if he'd anticipated any difficulty in the surgery.

I picked up a frayed copy of *Time* magazine and leafed through it. Everyone in town knew Dad because he'd been the director of the public library for thirty years. Dad was respected in our town, and he'd get the best care it had to offer. Anyway, it was too late to do anything different.

I yawned. Why did they keep the waiting room so warm? I felt myself begin to fade. I woke up, a thin string of drool dripping down the right side of my mouth. I wiped my chin and cheek with my palm, and looked around. No one seemed to have noticed. I wiped my palm on the leg of my jeans, stretched, and slumped back into the chair.

"Have a good nap?" Judie asked.

"Pretty good," I said.

"How long do you think it'll be?"

"Don't know," I said. "This guy's good?"

"Neal trusts him," Judie said.

"That's good," I said. Having a doctor you trust is important. As long as the guy's good.

"Feel free to doze some more," Judie said, looking up from her knitting.

"I may," I said, settling as comfortably as possible into the vinyl chair. I closed my eyes. Sleeping was better than worrying.

"Wake up," I heard Dr. Gardner's voice. He chuckled. "I was the same way when I was a resident," he said to Judie.

I stood, blinking.

"It went well. I wedged out a section about this big." He held his finger and thumb about three inches apart. "The frozen sections show clean margins," he said. "The finals will be out in a couple of days."

Judie looked at me.

"It means we got it all," Dr. Gardner said. "The pathologists will have to look at their specimens for a couple of days before they'll read out a final report, but they can tell from the frozen sections that I got it all."

"Was it cancer?" Judie asked.

"Oh, yes," Dr. Gardner replied. "Non-invasive, so he won't need chemo or radiation therapy." He held his hands out to his sides, palms forward. "Surgical cure."

"Thank you," Judie said.

"Yes," I said. "Thanks." I felt a rush of gratitude for this man who'd cut the cancer from my father's chest.

"Any questions?" He looked from me to Judie.

"Not right now," Judie said.

"You sure?" He waited a second, then nodded. "Maybe you'll have some when I come around this afternoon to check on him."

In the recovery room, Dad looked at Judie and me, then closed his eyes. By the time they took him to his room, he was awake, but still sedated from his morphine pump. "You-all okay?" he asked Judie and me, his words slow.

"Yes," Judie said. "We came through it very well."

Dad smiled, and dozed back off.

I spent the day in his room, with trips to the bathroom, the hospital gift shop, and the cafeteria. I felt an enormous sense of relief, knowing Dad's cancer had been cut away, dropped into a stainless steel bowl, and passed off to the gloved hand of the circulating nurse. Now the small chunk of abnormal meat was spread out in thin slices under a pathologist's microscope.

It was a strange sensation, hearing the overhead pages for doctors, seeing nurses hurry down the hall, seeing Dad's IV set up: it was like being at work on the wards, except there wasn't anything I was supposed to be doing.

Early the next morning, Judie dropped me off at the airport. I was glad I could return to Pittsburgh without worry: Dad's surgeon had taken good care of him. Dr. Gardner had been competent, caring, and approachable. He'd seemed eager to explain things, to make sure we understood everything. I'd misjudged him: I'd let the arrogance I'd picked up at a large teaching hospital bias me against a skillful clinician. I hoped my misgivings hadn't been obvious.

As the airplane taxied from the gate, I leaned back and relaxed, reassured by the flight attendant's familiar recital of seatbelts and flotation devices. Dad's surgeon seemed to have an entirely different practice than the one for which I was preparing. His patients knew him and respected him. When they saw him around town, they'd want to lift up their shirts to show him their scars. I knew that Dr. Gardner would have his share of difficult patients, but I doubted that any of them would be as angry or combative as the patients who shot and stabbed their way into the trauma service.

When I applied to medical school, I thought of myself as empathic and caring, and expected this to carry me through the rough spots. Then, during medical school and residency, I began to trust the role I was taking on—the white coat, stethoscope, and training all contributed to a sense of professionalism that helped me get through stressful times. I felt as if I was getting the hang of being a doctor.

Remembering the last patient I had seen on the trauma service—the drunk—I was ashamed of my angry outburst. When I rushed to his stretcher to yell at him, my emotions had been fully engaged. They felt more true and real than the Hippocratic Oath or any smooth platitude about bedside manner. When he sobered up, he wouldn't remember that I had jammed my face so close to his that our noses almost touched.

But I remembered it.

PART TWO

MRS. KELLY

"It's not that bad." Mr. Kelly smiled. "I'm not even hurting now." He was a forty-two-year-old housepainter who'd been having dull, intermittent chest pain for two days. Three wires ran from under his patient gown to the monitor in the corner, where a fine green line bounced with each beat of his heart.

His wife shifted in her chair. A disposal box for contaminated needles jutted from the wall, next to her head. She leaned away from it, as if she wanted to scoot her chair over. A stainless steel supply rack hemmed her in on the other side.

"It was just a nagging little pain." He gestured toward his chest. His fingernails were square and stubby, trimmed close. They glowed pink against the white paint stuck to his cuticles.

"When you have the pain," I asked, "how long does it last?"

"I don't know." He looked at his wife, then back to me. "About ten, fifteen minutes."

"Did you tell him about your arm hurting?" The lines on her face showed concern, worry. Mrs. Kelly was a thin woman; she sat with her feet tucked beneath the chair and her hands held tightly together in her lap.

"It didn't hurt that bad." He rolled his left shoulder. "I might'a pulled it at work. You know, moving ladders and all."

Mrs. Kelly shook her head.

I asked him about the cardiac risk factors: he didn't know his cholesterol, he smoked about a pack a day, and his father had had a heart attack when he was in his late fifties. I wrote orders for the standard chest pain work-up: EKG, cardiac enzymes, chest X-ray, and routine labs. "When the results come back, I'll come and talk with you." I gave the chart to the secretary and went to see my next patient.

The EKG was done promptly, and was normal. The results of the blood work came back later, and I went to the dictation booth to review them. They were normal, too. Even so, in the evaluation of chest pain the symptoms and risk factors are more important than the tests. The safest thing to do would be to admit Mr. Kelly overnight to check his cardiac enzymes two more times.

When you have a heart attack, enzymes from the damaged heart tissue leak out into the blood. If we check the cardiac enzymes early in the process, the level might not have gotten over the threshold of "positive." We check subsequent levels, to catch any rise that may occur over time. That's why we admit patients for "serial enzymes."

Mr. Kelly didn't have a physician, so I called the doctor who was on call for unassigned patients, to arrange for an overnight admission.

In training, interns and residents work incessantly. To a bleary-eyed intern who's hoping to sneak off and take a nap at three o'clock in the morning, a call from the ER is never good news. It doesn't mean he has an opportunity to help someone. It doesn't mean he's getting a case he can learn from. It just means he's gotten screwed out of the few hours of sleep he'd hoped to steal.

When a patient needs to be admitted to a university hospital, the senior resident goes to the ER and checks on the patient. If an admission is unavoidable, the senior calls the intern, who comes down to do the history and physical and write the admission orders. If there's some doubt as to the necessity of an admission, the senior resident may put up a fight with the ER attending, and try to talk him into sending the patient home. Some of the senior residents never question the ER attending. They're called "sieves," because they let everyone in. Those who consistently argue against admissions are called "walls." Sieves are despised by interns. Walls are worshipped: they shield their interns by thinking of fifty different reasons every patient could be discharged. And they just seem *smarter* than the sieves.

This attitude is understandable when you consider the hallucinatory, sleepless fog of residency and the fact that they're young, still in training. Most physicians outgrow this attitude. Some though, even years out of training, seem to take pride in being a wall, and sending people home from the ER.

I paged George Packard, the doctor on call for patients without a primary care physician. He's been in practice for years, and he's a wall. Proud of it. Has a cocky little walk he does if he discharges a patient the ER doc thought needed to be admitted. When we call him about one of his own patients, he'll try to talk us into sending them home. When he's on call for unassigned patients, he argues even more stubbornly. I wasn't looking forward to the call.

George returned the page, and listened to the history, physical exam, and labs.

"Sounds like he could go home."

"I don't know, George." I stared across the ER at a drunk, who was leaning further and further across the side rail of his stretcher. Blood dripped slowly from a laceration on his forehead. I covered the phone's mouthpiece. "Someone help that guy in room eight," I yelled. "He's about to fall." One of the health care techs strolled into the room and pushed the drunk back on the stretcher. "The guy has a strong family history and he's a smoker," I said into the phone. "Stoic guy, may be in denial. I think he's real, and he needs to come in."

"You think everyone needs to come in."

"This guy has a good story." The drunk had his head over the side rail and was looking at something on the floor.

"You're saying you think he's having a heart attack?"

"I'm saying I think he could have a plaque that hasn't ruptured yet."

"Didn't you just tell me he had a normal EKG, and negative enzymes?"

We both knew Mr. Kelly could be having a heart attack and initially have normal studies. That's why we admit patients for serial tests. "I don't know what to tell you, George." I shook my head. "Guy's dad had an MI in his fifties, he smokes a pack a day, and his pain is typical of ischemia."

"With a normal EKG, and negative enzymes after two *days* of pain. If anything was going to be positive, it already would've been. You know that."

"I think he needs to be admitted." I wished we had an equation we could apply to the problem. So many points for this risk factor, so many points for the other. But there isn't one. It all gets down to a judgment call, based on a few risk factors and very subjective symptoms. Pain versus pressure, discomfort versus pain. Is the patient exaggerating or minimizing his symptoms?

"I'd be glad to squeeze him in at the office, first thing in the morning. Do an accelerated outpatient work-up."

"I don't think he should go home tonight."

"Do you know how many hundreds of patients with bullshit chest pain we admit for every patient who has real disease? Or have any idea how much we spend, a year, on these worthless admissions? How much 'covering your ass' costs a year?"

"I'd love to talk about that sometime, but not right now." The drunk had given up whatever he'd been trying to do, and lay with his head half off the stretcher, passed out. "And we're not talking about 'covering my ass.' We're talking about a guy who needs to be admitted to rule out MI."

"If I come in, I'm just going to send him home."

"That'll be your decision."

"You're going to make the patient wait another two hours?" George's voice scaled upward with incredulity. "Just for me to come in and send him home? I'm offering to see him first thing in the morning. That's only fourteen hours from now."

Two paramedics stood in the hallway with an asthmatic patient on a stretcher, waiting for the charge nurse to tell them where to put him. The patient leaned forward, struggling with each breath. With the effort, muscles in his neck tightened into cords. His skin was gray, and shiny with sweat.

"George, the guy needs to come in."

"It's up to you." George was probably shrugging on the other end. "I'll come in, but it sounds like he can go home."

We didn't have a bed for the asthmatic and he was too sick to stay in the hall. No point in tying up a bed with Mr. Kelly if George was going to send him home. "You'll see my guy first thing in the morning?"

"Glad to." George's voice warmed up.

"Okay."

Mr. Kelly and his wife looked at me when I walked back into the cubicle. "Your EKG and labs are normal."

Mr. Kelly smiled, looked at his wife, then back to me. "That's great."

"I think we can let you go home."

"Great." Mr. Kelly grinned and nodded. His wife looked down at her hands.

"I've spoken with Dr. Packard, the doctor on call. He'll see you in the morning, in his office."

His wife didn't look up. I got the feeling that she wanted her husband to stay, but she didn't say anything.

"I think you'll be fine, but if you have any chest pain, come back immediately." I waited for them to respond. If either of them objected, I could call Packard back and tell him they were balking at going home. Mrs. Kelly didn't look up. Of course, I could call Packard back anyway and tell him to come to the ER and see the patient. Let *him* send the guy home.

I didn't.

Joanne, the charge nurse, had pulled a different patient into the hall, to make room for the asthmatic.

Lisa, one of the other nurses, was slapping the back of the patient's hand to find a vein in which to start an IV. "The line EMS put in blew." She didn't look up from her task. "I went ahead and started another breathing treatment."

"Good." I nodded to the patient, then, with my stethoscope, listened to the tight, high-pitched wheezing sounds of air barely moving in and out of his lungs. "You sound tight," I said to the man.

He nodded.

"Let's give him Solumedrol," I said to Lisa.

"Got it in my pocket." She looked up. "Can you hand me some tape?"

I tore two thin strips of tape and handed them to her.

"Thanks." She taped the IV in place. "There." She looked to me. "Portable X-ray?"

"Yup." With good nurses, an ER doc can get a lot done just by saying, "Yup." I saw Mr. Kelly and his wife walk past, toward the exit. I had an urge to call out, "Wait, let's check another EKG." But a repeat EKG would probably be normal too, and I would have felt foolish asking him to stay after I'd discharged him. I'd arranged a follow-up for the next morning. He'd be okay for fourteen hours.

"Paul," Lisa called. "This guy's looking sick."

I turned to the asthmatic, and forgot Mr. Kelly.

The next day when I started my shift, Joe Davidson, one of the other ER docs, was sitting in the dictation room. He was a runner, and looked like it. Tall, bony guy, with broad shoulders and no ass. He looked up from the chart he was working on. "Paul, you remember a guy named Kelly?"

My stomach felt queasy. "Guy with chest pain?"

"Yeah." Joe looked up from the chart he was holding. "He came back, about four thirty in the morning. Cardiac arrest."

I sat.

"You okay?"

"Yeah." I felt prickles in my scalp and down the back of my neck. I glanced at the trash can, afraid I might vomit. "He'd been having chest pain off and on. Didn't have any while he was here."

"I worked the code for at least thirty minutes before I called it," Joe said.

Mr. Kelly was dead.

Joe adjusted the stethoscope draped around his neck. "I looked over his EKG, and labs from when you'd seen him. They were normal."

"I know." I'd sent Mr. Kelly home, and now he's dead.

"It's gonna happen." Joe shook his head. "We can't admit every single chest pain that comes in. I would've done the same thing."

I still wanted to puke. "I had a bad feeling about him when I let him go."

Joe shrugged. "I sent home a guy last year. Came back a couple of hours later with ST segments like fucking Mount Everest." He was describing a classic EKG pattern of a heart attack.

"Did your guy make it?"

"Yeah," Joe said, "but that's not the point. I'd sent the guy home. I was just lucky."

He was trying to help me feel better. Every doctor has had a patient die as the result of a wrong judgment call, or a brief lapse of attention. It's inevitable when fallible people make mortal decisions. There are people who'll say, "This should *never* happen." And they're absolutely right. It shouldn't.

I struggled through the shift, oppressed by the knowledge that I'd sent Mr. Kelly home and that he'd died. Maybe if I'd paid attention to his wife, her unease would have prompted me to ask more questions. Maybe she would have told me something that would have made me insist on his admission to the hospital. But I'd looked Mr. Kelly in the eye and told him I thought he'd be okay, even though I had misgivings. There hadn't been enough hard data to convince George Packard to come in, and I'd not paid enough attention to an intuition, an uneasy feeling. I'd trusted Packard's judgment over mine.

In lectures, seminars, and magazine articles, malpractice lawyers tell you to never, never, never discuss a potential malpractice case. With anyone. The other side will ask if you'd discussed it, and have you make a list of names. Then they'll interview everyone, and find someone who remembers your admitting a mistake. In one class I listened to on cassette tape, the speaker told about a doc who'd confided in his wife about a mistake he'd made. Before the case went to court, the doc and his wife went through an acrimonious divorce. In the malpractice trial, his ex-wife took the stand against him with a vengeance. The class had roared with laughter at the poor schmuck's bad luck. You don't discuss the case, and you never, ever, apologize. To the malpractice lawyers, "I'm sorry" is just another way to say "I'm guilty."

The shift moved slowly, like a bad dream. Finally, it was over. I copied Mr. Kelly's phone number down on a scrap of paper before I left. When I got home, everyone was asleep. I wanted to wake Sally and tell her. But she was sleeping soundly, so I went downstairs and turned on the TV. A tall, handsome attorney with a very good toupee was on the screen. His voice was deep, and caring. "If you, or anyone in your family, has been injured by a doctor or a hospital, call me." A 1-800 number flashed on the screen. "We'll get the money *you deserve*." He somehow managed to mix enthusiasm with sadness in his voice. I vaguely wondered if Mrs. Kelly was at home alone, watching the same ad.

I clicked off the TV. I went to the kitchen, got a beer, went out on the front porch, and sat down on the steps. Two large magnolia trees shaded me from the street light. Mrs. Kelly was probably awake, too. Maybe sitting on her front porch looking out into the night, stunned by the emptiness she faced.

The next morning was my day off. After the kids were in school, I told Sally the whole story.

"Paul, there's no way you could've known he was going to die."

"His story was good enough to buy him an admission."

"No one's perfect." She shook her head. "I know it makes your job scary, but *everyone* is going to make mistakes."

"Yeah, but not like this." I rinsed my coffee cup. "Missing a fracture, or a urinary tract infection, stuff like that, sure, you're going to miss a few of them. But sending a guy home to die?" I felt the pain continue to build, of all places, in my chest. Maybe if I cried, I'd feel better.

"You didn't send anyone home to die." Sally sounded a little irritated. "You evaluated him, and made a decision." Simple as that. "No one expects you to be perfect."

"Even if I'd admitted him, he probably would have died."

"That's true." Sally nodded.

I leaned against the kitchen counter, my back to the sun coming through the kitchen window. "Must've been a huge MI, to have killed him so quickly." I needed to believe that Mr. Kelly would've died even if I'd admitted him, because nothing in my experience had prepared me for feeling so guilty. Up to the moment I found out Mr. Kelly had died, the possibility I could make an error of that magnitude had remained an abstraction, a theoretical possibility that wasn't grounded in personal experience. I'd been trained well and I was careful. I thought that if I was vigilant enough, I could practice indefinitely without seriously hurting anyone.

As a resident, I'd been shocked when Dr. Solters joked that he expected each of us to kill three patients in the process of becoming a doctor. At the time, a mistake that big was inconceivable. A few months later, I rotated through the cardiac care unit, and took care of Mrs. Mahoney, a seventy-one-year-old woman who'd had a heart attack. One night when I was on call, her blood pressure dropped precipitously. I was glad Dr. Putman was the cardiology fellow backing me up that night, because he was smart, decisive, and had sound judgment. He supervised us closely, and didn't resent getting out of bed to give us a hand. Dr. Putman decided that Mrs. Mahoney needed a Swan-Ganz catheter, which would allow us to record pressure readings from different areas inside her heart and lung. I enjoyed doing procedures, and had inserted several Swan-Ganz lines with Dr. Putman. We didn't anticipate any problems.

Nicole, one of the CCU nurses, helped me into my sterile gown and gloves, and then handed me the sterile equipment I'd be using. She and Dr. Putman watched as I carefully painted Mrs. Mahoney's upper chest and neck with orange antiseptic, and draped the area with sterile green drapes. I then stuck a long needle through the skin, and advanced it until it hit the collarbone. Mrs. Mahoney grunted in pain. "Sorry," I said. I withdrew the needle again, and angled it slightly lower. I was aiming for the large vein that runs just under the collarbone. If you angle your needle too steeply, you puncture the lung. The safe way to do it is to "walk" the needle down the collarbone. I advanced the needle again, until it hit bone a second time. She grunted again, and I apologized again. The third time I pushed the needle into her chest, dark red blood filled my syringe. I was where I wanted to be, in the vein. "Don't move," I told Mrs. Mahoney, as I threaded a long, softly springy wire through the needle, and into the vein. I withdrew the needle, leaving the wire sticking up through the skin. Using the wire as a guide, I pushed a white plastic tube about the size of a small soda straw through the skin, under the collarbone, and into the vein. I sewed it securely to the skin of her chest, to keep it from being accidentally pulled free. All of these steps went without a hitch. I leaned back, took a deep breath, and let it out. So did Dr. Putman.

"Ready to float the Swan?" he asked.

I nodded to Dr. Putman. "The hard part's over," I told Mrs. Mahoney, "but you still need to hold still."

"Okay," she said, in a quiet voice.

After Nicole and I calibrated the equipment, I slipped a fine, supple catheter through the white plastic tube and into the vein under her collarbone. I advanced the catheter further, until it was in her heart, and then inflated the tiny balloon at the end of the catheter by injecting air into the appropriate port. The catheter was swept along with the flow of blood, out into the vessels of her lungs. We followed its progress by watching the pressure changes on the monitor screen as the catheter threaded its way through the chambers of the heart and out into the pulmonary arteries.

"Good," Dr. Putman said. "Let the balloon down and re-wedge it to be sure."

I nodded. Dr. Putman was meticulous, which is one of the reasons I liked working under his supervision. I let down the balloon. Nicole recorded the pressures, and I gently reinflated the balloon. Nicole nodded. "Yup. They're the same."

Dr. Putman grinned. "Good job."

Nicole said, "Smooth."

I smiled behind my sterile mask, and began to remove the sterile paper sheet covering Mrs. Mahoney's chest.

Mrs. Mahoney shuddered, then coughed up a huge mouthful of blood.

"Damn." Dr. Putman went to the head of the bed. "Mrs. Mahoney?"

She heaved out another gush of blood, then another.

What had I done? I took a small step away from the bed.

"What's her pressure?" Dr. Putman asked Nicole.

"I palpate it at 50." She dropped the BP bulb. "You want fluids?"

"Yeah, give her a liter wide open." He turned to me. "How much resistance did you meet when you inflated the second time?"

"None." I shook my head rapidly. "It went easy."

"You must've blown open a pulmonary artery." He frowned and crossed his arms. "But how'd the blood get from her interstitium into her airway?"

I stood without moving.

Mrs. Mahoney chugged out another mouthful of blood.

"We're going to have to tube her," Dr. Putman told me. He turned to Nicole. "Call for O-negative blood, and hang Dopamine."

I went for the airway box. Usually I enjoyed intubating people, but this time blood kept pouring up out of her trachea. My hands shook so much I could barely get the tube in. A respiratory therapist arrived just as I secured the tube in place, and took over squeezing the bag that pushed air into Mrs. Mahoney's lungs. I stepped away from the stretcher, and stripped off my bloody gloves.

I watched, stunned, as Dr. Putman ran the code. Nicole did chest compressions until she tired out, then another nurse took over. Dr. Putman told me to call Mrs. Mahoney's husband, and ask him to come in, but not tell him why. We'd explain it when he got there. After about an hour, Dr. Putman told them to stop CPR. Mrs. Mahoney's husband was in the CCU waiting room.

Dr. Putman did the talking. He said that Mrs. Mahoney had begun to bleed as we were doing a procedure. I sat quietly, glad I wasn't the one having to tell Mr. Mahoney that his wife was dead. Dr. Putman asked permission to do an autopsy, to see what had caused the bleeding, but Mr. Mahoney said that his wife had been through enough so he refused.

When he said that, I felt my burden begin to lighten. Without an autopsy, who could say for certain that I'd killed Mrs. Mahoney? Maybe she had something else going on, and it was just coincidental that the blood started gushing out right after I reinflated the balloon. And I still couldn't figure out how that much blood would get from the pulmonary artery into the airways. But even though my brain couldn't resolve how I'd killed Mrs. Mahoney, my body was certain that I had. My fingers had held the syringe and my thumb had gently pressed the plunger. Fourteen years later, it's still a visceral memory. But Dr. Putman had walked me, step by step, into the disaster. A teacher I respected and trusted had stood at the bedside with me. If we'd killed Mrs. Mahoney, I could tell myself, it was Dr. Putman's fault, not mine . . .

But I was the only one standing at the end of his stretcher

when I told Mr. Kelly and his wife that he'd be okay. I'd sent him out and he'd come back dead. I sat at the kitchen table, replaying the scene of Mr. Kelly and his wife shuffling down the hall in the ER, wishing I could rewind it all, call out to them and tell them that I'd changed my mind, that I'd admit him to the hospital.

The phone rang. It was Ken Anderson, one of the guys in our group. He's been an ER doc for twenty years. He has graying hair, a calm voice, and never seems to hurry. Even when the ER is rocking, Ken looks like he just strolled off the golf course. I don't know how he does it: each month we get a report on how many patients we see each hour, and Ken's numbers are consistently good, but he rarely seems perturbed, and I've never seen him look rushed. "Paul," he said, "I was going to drop by if you're around."

"Sure," I said. "You know our address?"

"Yeah," he said, "I'm about a block away."

"Okay." I hung up. "That was Ken," I told Sally. "He's coming over."

"It'll be good to talk with him," she said. "Why don't I go work in the yard some, give you guys some space." She stepped forward for a quick hug, then walked out the back door.

I went to the bathroom, then peered at my face in the mirror, hoping I didn't look as vulnerable as I felt. I also hoped I wasn't in trouble with the hospital, or the group of ER docs I worked with. I felt vaguely nauseated again.

Ken knocked on the door, and I let him in. He followed me back to the kitchen.

"I was just about to make a pot of coffee," I said.

"Sounds good." He sat in the chair at the end of the kitchen table.

"Are you here about Mr. Kelly?" I rinsed the basket of the coffeemaker, and put in a clean filter.

"Yeah."

I turned to look at Ken. "I feel terrible."

"You should," he said. "The man died."

I turned back around, hoping I hadn't outwardly flinched. Neither of us spoke as I silently counted the scoops of coffee. I dropped the scoop back into the coffee jar, and closed it.

"And good doctors," Ken continued, "are bothered when one of their patients dies."

Ken still thought I was a good doctor? I felt a wave of gratitude and relief. I put the coffeepot under the basket and punched the button to start the brewing. "I feel like I killed the guy."

"Whoa," Ken said. "Back up a minute. You didn't kill anybody. You're not even sure of the cause of death."

"Guy comes in with chest pain, comes back dead?" I turned to face Ken. "Doesn't seem like rocket science to me."

"Okay, say the man died of a heart attack. No matter how careful, how smart, or how compulsive you are, eventually you're going to make a mistake."

"Yeah, I know." I sat down in the chair at the other end of the table. "Missing something really obscure, or something so rare no one else would've picked it up either." I shrugged. "To me, that wouldn't be so hard to live with. But sending home a patient who's having a heart attack?"

"Paul, we can't admit every single patient who comes in with chest pain." Ken shook his head. "It's impossible. The hospital wouldn't hold them all." He looked over his shoulder at the coffeepot. "I think it's ready."

I got up and poured us each a cup.

"I'm just glad it was you, and not me."

"Thanks, pal." I tried to chuckle.

"What can I say?" He sipped his coffee. "Luck of the draw who picks up what chart."

"Ken, have you ever sent someone home and they came back dead?"

He carefully set his cup down, and gently rapped the table with his knuckles. "Knock on wood."

I wrapped my hands around the mug of coffee to feel the warmth.

"But, Paul," he said, "it's going to happen. It's like driving a car. No matter how careful you are, someday you're going to glance down at the radio to change stations, look up, and there's a car right in front of you. You've had a clean driving record for thirty years, you're a model citizen, and *boom*. You've plowed into some little old lady's Cadillac." He shook his head. "I'm not saying you made a mistake with this guy, but even good drivers have accidents."

"How do you do it?"

"Do what?"

"Keep on making life and death decisions, knowing that you're fallible."

"Paul, I don't make life and death decisions." He carefully put his coffee cup on the table. "I make medical decisions." He gave a slight shrug. "I work as carefully as I can, but it's not up to me who lives and who dies."

I stared at Ken's face.

"That's God's department."

Okay.

"Do you know what happens when a patient dies?"

"Yeah," I said. "The doc feels like shit."

"That's not what I mean." Ken looked away, then back at me. "We know a lot about how cells live. And we can describe, down at the molecular level, what happens when a cell dies: membranes break down, oxidative phosphorylation fails, hydrogen ions accumulate in the cytoplasm, all that stuff. But do we really know why people die?"

I couldn't see what he was getting at.

"Say someone comes in with a pulmonary embolism. We understand the pathophysiology: hypoxia, hypotension, acidosis, et cetera." He paused. "And we know how to intervene."

I nodded.

"But when a patient dies, what happens?" He raised his eyebrows. "I mean, one moment they're alive, and the next, they're not. You've felt it. We all have. Something's happened, and we don't know what it is. Sure, we can trace out the failures of the circulatory system, and we can get EEGs for brain activity." Ken shook his head. "But the fundamental thing of death itself it something we still don't understand."

"So?" I said.

"So, I look at each EKG as carefully as I can, and interview each patient as carefully as I can, and I make decisions as carefully as I can. Then I do my job and I let God do his." Ken held his hands out, palms up. "How can we possibly claim the credit for success, or take the blame for failure, in a process we don't really understand?"

I shrugged.

"Paul, you and I both know that you did your best for that man." Ken shook his head. "That's all any of us can do."

When I'd first started working in Durham, I'd been surprised by how much I liked talking with Ken. In so many ways, we're polar opposites: He's a conservative Republican. He wears knit shirts and khaki pants on his days off. He belongs to two country clubs, one here in Durham, one at his beach house. He thinks Rush Limbaugh is smart. I'd always thought of Ken as someone with useful answers to questions about buying stocks or avoiding taxes, but I hadn't thought he'd be the one to say something that would help me deal with Mr. Kelly's death.

Ken stood, and took his coffee mug to the kitchen counter. "Give my love to Sally."

"I will. Tell Barbara I said hey."

Ken rinsed his cup, and left it in the sink. "You're going to feel bad for a while," he said. "That's okay. Just keep feeling bad. You'll eventually feel better."

We walked to the front door.

"When do you work again?"

"Day after tomorrow."

"See you then." He stuck out his hand. "Paul, you're a good doctor."

"Thanks." We shook hands, and he left. I felt my eyes fill, and hoped Ken hadn't noticed. It must have been awkward for him to come by and talk with me, and I didn't want to go all gushy on him. I felt as though being a good father, or a good husband, or a good man, was a hollow success if I wasn't a good doctor as well. I was glad that Ken thought I was a good doctor. I just wished I felt that way.

After Ken drove away, I walked outside. It was a bright, sunny day. I sat in a wicker chair, and wondered if prayer would offer some relief. I prayed silently, but felt a need for something more physical and real than closing my eyes and thinking about God. My palms were sweaty. I wiped my hands on my jeans, and looked out at the street. The sun was still bright, the porch was still in the shade. A woman walked past, a dog tugging on the leash. I closed my eyes. "God, forgive me. And be with Mrs. Kelly, and their kids, if they have any." I took a deep breath. "Comfort them. And let them know I did the best I could, and I'm sorry." I opened my eyes. No change.

Maybe I should talk with Karen, or James. They're our pastors, at the Pilgrim United Church of Christ. Sally grew up in that denomination and a pastor from her parents' church had performed the ceremony when we'd gotten married. When Sally and I had kids, we started going to the Pilgrim UCC in Durham. The folks there seem like Unitarians, only less embarrassed to be called Christians. We went to Sunday School and church almost every Sunday I was off duty. I went to the Adult Bible Study Class. Matthew, my Sunday School teacher, was a law professor at Duke. Worked with Janet Reno on some legal stuff, worked with Al Gore on the problem about the use of the telephone at the White House. I felt lucky to discuss Christianity with such a smart crowd. So much of Christianity in the South seems anti-intellectual: TV preachers sputtering about sin and pleading for money, telephone numbers flashing on the screen. I've always felt like a second-rate Christian, insufficiently saved, with inadequate fervor. At the same time, I feel the Bible drawing me back, particularly the four Gospels. I believe there are answers there. And a model of grace. A model of how I can live.

I went inside and called Karen. She said I could come right over. I changed jeans, splashed my face, and drove to our church, a brick building that's mostly roofline, tucked in among a thick stand of trees that shields it from the traffic on the street.

I knocked on her office door and Karen let me in. The bookshelves lining the wall were filled with paperbacks, probably texts from divinity school. Light filtered in through windows looking out into woods. She got up from behind her desk, and gestured to an upholstered chair. Another chair faced mine. She pulled it toward mine a little, and sat. "Are you okay?"

I nodded. "Yeah, basically." I told her the story. "I feel so bad. So *guilty*." I looked at the floor, then back to Karen. "You know, in the Bible, it says if we want God to forgive us for something we did to someone else, we should first ask that person's forgiveness? Something about leaving the gift on the altar, straightening out the problem, then coming back."

Karen nodded.

"I want to call Mrs. Kelly and tell her I'm sorry."

"It'll be a tough call to make." Karen was looking me in the eyes.

"Not as hard as walking around feeling as bad as I do now."

"Maybe."

"I don't know if I'm wanting to call Mrs. Kelly to make her feel better, or to make *myself* feel better."

"And?"

"It's probably a little of both."

Karen waited.

"Do I have the right to call Mrs. Kelly, just to make myself feel better?"

"Paul," Karen's voice scaled down several tones. "It's all right for you to want forgiveness." She shook her head. "God doesn't want you to carry guilt and pain around every step of your life."

I didn't feel anything in my chest loosen up or any burden lighten. But I caught a glimmer of the possibility. I thanked her.

When I got home, I looked at the phone number on the scrap of paper.

Sally walked into the kitchen. She was sweaty, from mowing the yard. "How did it go with Karen?"

"I'd hoped I would feel better."

Sally smiled. "You look a little better."

"I think I'll call Mrs. Kelly." I walked to the sink and got a glass of water. "Tell her I'm sorry."

Sally hugged me from behind. I could feel the damp of her shirt.

"If I call Mrs. Kelly, and it goes to court, they'll make a big deal about me calling her to apologize."

Sally shrugged.

"If the award goes past my malpractice coverage, it could come out of our pockets."

"So what. It'll probably never happen." She shrugged again. "And if it does: Fuck 'em."

If nothing else, I'd married well.

Sally pulled back to look at me. "You should call her. You may feel better." She hugged me again. "I'll be on the front porch."

Mrs. Kelly picked up the phone on the third ring.

"This is Paul Austin, I'm the doctor who took care of your husband the first time he came to the emergency room."

"Oh."

"I'm calling to say I'm sorry." I paused. "I'm sorry your husband died."

She didn't answer.

"Mrs. Kelly?"

"I'm here."

I waited. "If you have any questions, or concerns . . ."

There was another pause. "Why did you send my husband home?"

The question thumbed me in the chest. "I thought he would be okay." I took a breath. "I was wrong. And I'm sorry."

She didn't answer.

I waited.

She didn't say anything.

I looked down at the crumbs on the floor. "If there's anything you want to say to me . . ." I winced at the accusations she might unleash, but held a glimmer of hope she'd say she forgave me.

"I've got nothing to say to you right now."

I gave her my home phone number, and told her if she ever had anything to say, or any other questions, I'd be glad to talk with her.

We hung up.

I didn't feel any better. And it seemed that Mrs. Kelly didn't feel any better, either. But at least I'd said I was sorry.

I walked out to the front porch.

Sally looked up from her novel. "How did it go?"

I sat in the chair next to her. "She didn't have anything to say to me."

Sally closed her novel, keeping her place with her finger.

"I didn't really expect her to flat-out forgive me, but I'd hoped for something." Glints of sunlight reflected off the hard, waxy leaves of the magnolia tree in front of the porch. I could barely make out the pitted gray bark of the trunk through the dark openings between the leaves. "*Some* human contact."

"It's early." Sally patted my knee.

"Did I call too soon?" I felt my dismay grow heavier. Had I added to Mrs. Kelly's pain, just to ease my own?

"Probably not." Sally shook her head. "But who knows when you should've called? She might've been sitting at her kitchen table just now, wondering why the ER doctor hadn't even bothered to call." Sally turned in her chair to face me. "At least now she knows her husband was important to the doctor. Paul, you've done everything you could—you saw the guy, did all the tests, thought about it, and told him to come back if he had more pain." She held up a finger with each point. "Nobody's perfect."

I nodded that I'd heard, and I understood what she was saying. But I wanted relief from the guilt I felt, to somehow snap out of it—to learn my lesson and move on. It's hard to know how guilty one should feel if, in good faith, one harms another. How does one "get over" a mistake that cost another person's life?

SPLINTERS

I MANAGED to work my next few shifts without killing anyone, but every decision seemed to vibrate with danger. Each time I signed my name at the bottom of a chart to discharge a patient, I had a superstitious fear that, like Mr. Kelly, he'd be rushed back to the ER in an ambulance, with a burly paramedic doing chest compressions.

Even the simple cases became tricky. A guy who'd twisted his ankle playing basketball had minimal tenderness and no swelling. The X-ray was normal, but I couldn't be 100 percent positive there wasn't a subtle fracture I was missing, so I splinted his ankle in plaster. My indecision meant he'd be hobbling around on crutches until he saw the orthopedist in a couple of weeks. At best he'd be taking all his baths with his foot wrapped up in a plastic bag and his lower leg dangling outside of the tub—at worst, he could fall after getting tangled up in his crutches as he lurched down the stairs of his apartment. I hated to think of that, but I really hated the idea of *missing* something.

A patient with a simple chest cold insisted on an X-ray to make sure she didn't have pneumonia. The film didn't show anything, but what if I was missing a subtle infiltrate? Probably best just to put her on antibiotics. But what if she had an allergic reaction to the unnecessary antibiotics, and rushed back in with her eyes puffy, making tight squeaky noises through her airway that was swelling shut? Every patient offered an infinite regression of second-guesses, and I felt more like a third-year medical student than an experienced attending physician in an ER. Of course, a patient with chest pain was the worst. I was afraid I'd telegraph my insecurity, so I tried to modulate my voice to a calm and confident register.

It took a month or so, but eventually I could introduce myself without the hollow, queasy fear that I might fail a person who trusted me. I could do it, but as I finished each shift, I was anxious and jittery.

At home I tried not to think about Mr. Kelly, or to wonder about the other mistakes I might have made but hadn't yet heard about. One weekday morning I slept late, then padded downstairs to the kitchen, grateful for a few days off to recuperate after working four late evening shifts in a row. It's hard to work in an urban ER for more than three or four days in a row because the pace is so intense. You can get overloaded to the point that you're caring less, which makes you more likely to make a mistake. For the previous four nights the paramedics had been banging away at us non-stop, bringing in patient after patient. Our waiting room and hallways had remained full of bored, tired, angry people.

I needed a break.

Sally sat at the table, leafing through the newspaper. She leaned forward to give me a hug around the hips. "Coffee?" she asked, as she got a mug from the cabinet.

"Yes, please." I was glad to have four days off coming up, and hoped to let the tension drain out of my system so I could enjoy them.

"Where are the kids?" I asked.

"Watching *Sesame Street*." Sally set a steaming mug of coffee in front of me. "I'm glad you could sleep late." She added a small dollop of milk.

I took a sip. "Me too." I yawned, and looked at the clock radio on the kitchen counter—10:17. I'd left work about midnight and had finally gotten to sleep by two. I counted on my fingers—I'd gotten eight solid hours of sleep. I yawned again, looking forward to a day of hanging around the house without anything pressing to do. No one calling my name on the squawking overhead speakers, or having a seizure in room 6. No impatient family members standing in the hallway glaring at me.

I could read, doze off, wake up, then read some more. Or I could stretch out in bed for a real nap, or maybe fish on the banks of the Eno River with a cane pole and a bunch of worms. I'd been holding the stress in tightly, careful not to blow up at anyone. Now I could let the sun bake it out of me, and let the tension slowly release into the warm spring air.

"Cereal?" Sally asked.

"I'll get some in a minute," I said. I read *Doonesbury*, *Blondie*, and *Peanuts*, mindfully skipping *Garfield* and the other comics that irritated me. After working in ERs for several years, I was finally getting the hang of dealing with stress. All I had to do was keep my guard up and clamp down on my emotions until I got the chance to decompress. Then I could let the pressure out slowly, like easing open a bleed-off valve on an air compressor. That morning was a perfect example.

I took the editorial page to the bathroom and gave myself a little diagnostic test. Could I read the letters to the editor without getting irritated? I scanned the hostile letters from my fellow Durham citizens without a single beat of vexation.

After washing my hands, I started back to the kitchen for a bowl of cereal, enjoying the coolness of the linoleum floor on my bare feet. The door to the kitchen was closed. I turned the doorknob, expecting to walk right through. Instead, I stubbed my toe against the door because it wouldn't open. *Damn.* Previous owners had attached a barrel bolt to the door leading from our kitchen to the mudroom, half-bath, and laundry room. They'd also drilled a quarter-inch hole into the trim of the doorframe, into which the barrel bolt could slide. The barrel bolt must've been engaged. Must've been Sarah, playing during a break from her TV show. I let go of my foot and knocked on the door. "Sally?"

No answer.

I knocked again. "Sally?" A little louder.

I considered going out the back door and coming back in the front door, but I didn't feel like hopping barefoot through the dew-soaked grass. "Sally?" *Why had she just wandered off after letting Sarah lock the door?*

I grabbed the doorknob and rattled the door.

I felt a hot flush of anger. I shook the door harder. *Fuck this.* I smacked my shoulder against the door and popped it open. A chunk of doorframe as long as my hand went spinning into the kitchen, torn loose by the engaged barrel bolt. *There. Door open, problem solved.*

My heart was beating hard. My vision was clearer, sharper than before. The kids' cereal bowls stacked next to the sink, the morning sun's shadows in the folds of the curtains, the fine shards of wood scattered around the larger piece on the floor, all stood out in clear and sharp relief.

I listened for Sally, but heard nothing. Must've gone upstairs. I bent over to examine the damage to the doorframe, feeling a flush of shame. Flecks of white paint had splintered off, revealing the barn red enamel I'd painted over when we moved in. I picked up the long, jagged piece of wood and placed it on the kitchen counter.

My hand shook as I poured my cereal and milk. I leafed through the grocery store ads. I turned and looked at the doorframe, then back to my cereal.

Sally walked through the kitchen with a laundry basket of whites. She stopped at the splintered jamb. "What happened?" Her voice sounded concerned, the way it did when John had limped into the house with a skinned knee, or Sarah ran toward her after a bee sting. She set the laundry basket on the floor and leaned over, lightly running her fingers across the doorframe.

"Door was locked."

She stared at me, then at the splinters at her feet, then back at me.

"I must be feeling more stress than I thought." I looked down at my toe. "Sorry."

"Paul," she said. "You need to do something."

"Soon as I finish breakfast." I looked up. "A little wood glue, a few brads . . ." I knew she wasn't talking about the doorframe. She wanted me to get therapy. She was a psychiatric nurse, and her father had been a psychiatrist. She thought everyone needed therapy.

She paused.

"Some sandpaper, a little paint."

"Okay." Her tone said she knew I'd purposefully misunderstood her, but she wasn't going to argue about it again. Sally carried a basketful of dirty clothes into the laundry room.

The initial step of patching the door took twenty minutes. The splintered ends of the large piece meshed perfectly with the broken edges of the doorframe. I was afraid that the wood might split along the grain, so I drilled tiny little holes for each skinny little brad, before I tapped each one gently home. The smaller splinters held with wood glue alone.

As soon as the glue dried, I sanded the patch job, and puttied the remaining cracks smooth. That afternoon I sat in the sun, reading Wallace Stegner's *The Angle of Repose*. Midafternoon, I sanded again, and brushed on some thirty-minute primer, then painted over it.

As soon as the paint was dry, the damage was almost invisible under the doorframe's smooth and shiny surface.

TUCKER PUT HIS GUN TO HIS HEAD

Barry, the senior paramedic, was at the head of the gurney as they wheeled into the trauma bay of our ER. "This guy shot himself," Barry said. "It's a mess. A goddamn mess." One of the other paramedics pumped on the guy's chest while a firefighter fumbled to undo the yellow straps securing him to their gurney.

Barry wiped his forehead with the back of his wrist, keeping the blood on his gloved hand from touching his face. "He stood there in the kitchen, told his mom, 'I'm going to shoot myself,' and then, *boom*." Barry snorted, and shook his head. "Couldn't intubate him so we've been using the bag ventilator. Sorry, Doc."

"No problem," I said. "Let's move him over to our stretcher." I was working the 3:00–11:00 P.M. shift. We'd been scrambling to catch up, but patients filled every cubicle and lay on stretchers lining the hallways. A demented woman from a nursing home screeched incoherent complaints from room 27, and next to the nursing station, a man slumped forward in a wheelchair, mumbling loudly into his lap.

Barry raised his voice and counted: "One, two, three." The paramedics and firefighters hefted the man over to our bed. They pulled their narrow gurney out of the room, trailing a monitor lead on the floor.

The nurses snapped cardiac monitor wires onto the man's chest and wrapped a blood pressure cuff around his arm while I tried to slip a plastic tube down his throat and into his windpipe. His head jostled with the rhythm of chest compressions, and blood and vomit welled up into the back of his mouth. I tried to clear it out with a suction catheter, but it kept getting plugged with bits of yellow-white cheesy stuff. "Bag him up some," I said to the respiratory therapist. "I'm going to try to suction him with straight tubing; maybe it won't get clogged."

As she squeezed the bag to force air into his lungs, a flatulent sound and a fine red mist came from a bullet hole just above his ear. "Damn," the respiratory therapist said, "what's that?"

I stood and stared, perplexed by the small bloody geyser coming out the side of the man's head with each squeeze of the Ambu-bag. Then it occurred to me. The bullet must have angled down through his skull and brain and then through the roof of his mouth. I pulled the face piece off, and looked into his mouth. Sure enough, there was a jagged hole through the soft palate.

I looked over at the paramedics. "How long's he been down?"

Barry looked at his watch. "Twenty-five, thirty minutes."

"Did he ever have a pulse?"

Barry shook his head.

"This isn't a survivable injury." I looked around the room, at each person. "Unless anyone has any other ideas, I'm going to call it." It is a team effort, and I like to give everyone a chance to speak up before ending a resuscitation.

Beth looked at the clock on the wall. "Time of death 07:52."

Nurses seem to recognize the futility of doomed efforts before physicians do. Beth spoke clearly, and loudly, so everyone would document the same time of death.

"Good job, everybody," I said. "This guy was just too dead." I looked at the paramedics standing in the doorway, watching. "Who tried to intubate him?"

Barry raised his hand, and looked at the floor. "I couldn't see anything from all the blood and vomit." He looked up at me. "We decided to load and go."

"You did the right thing." I stripped off my gloves and the paper disposable gown. "Bits of brain kept clogging the suction catheter." I clapped his shoulder. "You were right to scoop and run."

He looked at his feet. "Thanks."

"Sure." I looked down the hallway. "The family coming?"

"I think his sister will." Barry looked up. "The mother probably won't. She's old, shook up pretty bad."

"Do we know the guy's name?"

"Tucker. Tucker Walton."

"He was dead when he hit the floor." I didn't want Barry to feel bad about not being able to intubate the guy.

Barry looked down at his feet again and nodded.

I asked Beth to tell me when the sister was in the Family Room, and then went to the nurses' station to call the coroner and began filling out the paperwork.

I usually hate filling out forms, but the blanks on the death certificate offered a refuge from my emotions. The freakish red geyser coming from the hole above the man's ear had surprised me, but it wasn't as disturbing as the thought of a warm, slack body sprawled out on a linoleum floor. A dead body on a stretcher is just that—a dead body on a stretcher. It's a simple physical fact. But a man lying on his mother's kitchen floor is more complicated; he's a person. I needed to keep things simple. Charts of the still-living were stuffed, two to a slot, in the rack under the clock in the nurses' station. I still had three more hours to work.

I clicked my pen and wrote Mr. Walton's name in careful block print, at the top of the form. In the line listing "Cause of death," I wrote: "Gunshot wound to head—Self-inflicted." Like most males, his suicide attempt had been violent, and effective. When men try to kill themselves, it's usually by shooting, hanging, or jumping off a bridge. Women tend to overdose on drugs, or try to drown themselves. Women try to kill themselves three to four times more often than men, but men are three to four times more likely to succeed.

The next line on the form read: "As a consequence of." It's for listing contributing factors. For example, if Mr. Walton had died from a heart attack, I'd write, "Myocardial infarction" in the first line, and list "Coronary artery disease" as a contributing factor. But he hadn't died of a heart attack. He'd killed himself, and I didn't know why. He probably had a psychiatric history, since 90 percent of suicides are related to a mood disorder or other psychiatric illness. It's a large number, which has grim implications for people with depression, but more than 95 percent of people with psychiatric disorders *don't* commit suicide. Another likely contributing factor is alcohol, since it's involved in 64 percent of suicide attempts, but a death certificate isn't the place to write down guesses. I skipped the "consequence" line.

I saw my first suicide when I was in my early twenties and I was a firefighter in my hometown. Late one Saturday night, it could've been early Sunday morning, I was asleep in my bunk when all of the lights flashed on and the bells clanged. The overhead speaker blared in the bored southern monotone of the dispatcher: "Attention, Engine Five, respond to Twelve-forty-three Maple Leaf Road. Self-inflicted gunshot wound to the head." We all sprang from our beds, hearts pounding from the adrenaline surge of being jerked into wakefulness so abruptly. In one motion, we swung our feet off the sides of our bunks and into the black rubber boots and yellow canvas pants. We ran down the hall to the fire engine, where we put on our turn-out coats and helmets, and climbed up into our seats. Doug Ramsey and I rode in jump seats behind the captain and the driver. The diesel motor roared between us. I looked over at Doug. He blinked, like a kid who'd just woken up in a place he didn't recognize.

I didn't feel the excitement I usually felt on the way to a fire. Most of us hated medical calls. When we pulled up to a burning building, we were sure of our roles. There's a physical thrill in doing even the simplest task when you're putting out a fire: jumping from the truck and dragging an inch-and-a-half-thick line toward a house with flame blossoming from the windows, feeling the rough canvas hose spring and lurch as it fills with water. And we were good at it. But when we were on a medical call, standing in someone else's bedroom, watching an old man sweat with pain, we were never sure what to do. We'd put an oxygen mask on the patient's face and hook him up to a cardiac monitor, and stare at the wavy green line, no clue as to what it meant. Then we'd stand there feeling clumsy in our yellow coats and hats, wishing the paramedics would hurry up.

Engine Five rumbled through the empty streets, the ride seeming quiet without the siren and air horn. Our red lights flashed across the fronts of darkened houses like a pale red strobe. The cold night air whipped past us, and I shivered inside my coat. We pulled up to a small brick ranch house where a woman stood on the front porch, screaming. Doug and I clambered off the truck and ran up the front steps to the porch. The woman screamed over and over, a high, shrieking wail I couldn't understand. She didn't seem to see us as we bounded up the steps. I eased past her, into the warm air of the living room, where a man reclined in a tan vinyl La-Z-Boy. His feet were crossed at the ankles, as if he were relaxing, or perhaps he'd dozed off while reading the newspaper. His right hand rested in his lap, a large, western-style handgun pointing lazily toward the floor. The wall behind was splashed with red. His hair was long and stringy. Blood dripped from a curl coming down beside his face. His eyes were half closed.

I stood and stared. Then I remembered the CPR classes with Resusci-Annie. I walked over to him and patted his shoulder. Just like I'd learned in class, I loudly said, "Are you okay? Are you okay?"

Doug stood behind me and looked over my shoulder. "Is he . . . ?"

"I think so." I felt his neck for a pulse. There wasn't one. I prodded him again, and his head lolled to the side.

Justin, our captain, came in, cautiously looking around the room. He walked up beside me, and stared at the man in the chair. "Is he dead?"

"Yeah, I think so." I pointed at the head and wall. "Looks like he shot himself in the head."

Justin called headquarters on his walkie-talkie. We stood in the living room, shifting from one foot to the other. We weren't paramedics. This wasn't what we were trained, or inclined, to do. We were firefighters. Guys who liked to crawl into burning buildings and spray water into the fire. Guys with families and part-time jobs, guys who liked to keep the grass at the firehouse trimmed just so. We weren't prepared to stand around a man who'd splattered his brains against a wall.

I became aware again of the woman shrieking on the front porch. I went out to see if she was injured. She stood in a sheer nightgown, goose bumps on her arms. Her breath smelled of too much bourbon. She kept shrieking. I couldn't make out the words. I took off my turn-out coat, made of a coarse, yellow canvas with a thick quilt lining, and put it around her shoulders. She faced me and looked directly into my eyes. Clearly and slowly she whispered, "He shot hisself." A thin string of mucous hung from her nose. She started wailing again, and I understood what she'd been shrieking all along. "He shot hisself he shot hisself he shot hisself he shot hisself." She leaned against me, resting her head on my shoulder, which soon felt damp from her tears. A person was silhouetted in a window in the house across the street.

The paramedics finally arrived and hustled into the room with their boxes of equipment. I stood on the porch and let the drunk woman slump against me and cry, feeling awkward in my T-shirt and yellow fireman's helmet. A few minutes later, the paramedics walked back to their truck, now without any urgency, to get the stretcher to haul the dead man to the morgue at the hospital. After they'd bundled him into the ambulance and closed the back door, one of the paramedics led the woman to the unit, opened the front door, and helped her in.

As the ambulance pulled off, the window across the street went dark. I pulled on my turn-out coat, glad to have the warmth. As we rode back to the station, I was comforted by the loud rumble of the diesel engine in the fire truck, but the woman's perfume still lingered along with the familiar smoky smell of my coat.

I'd just completed the death certificate when Beth came over. "The sister's in the Family Room," she said.

I looked up. "Anyone else?"

"No, just her."

"Let me go to the bathroom; then we'll go talk to her."

I went to the bathroom, splashed my face, made sure there wasn't any blood on my scrubs, and came back out to the nurses' station.

Beth was typing her nurse's notes into the computer. "Just a sec." She finished her note, logged off the computer, and stood.

"Can you stay with her until someone shows up?" I didn't want to leave the sister by herself, but didn't want to get stuck too long in the Family Room while there were still so many patients to be seen. You never know if someone in the waiting room is taking Tums for their "indigestion" while a blood clot is occluding a coronary artery. Beth was good with patients and their families, and would comfort Tucker's sister so I could spring free to see more patients.

"I'll sit with her," Beth said.

We walked into the Family Room. A thin woman was sitting with her knees together and her hands in her lap. Her face was calm.

I sat down in the chair next to hers and introduced myself. "You are his . . ."

"Sister," she answered.

"Do you know what happened today?"

"Tucker's been talking about shooting himself for years," she said in a soft voice. "Today, he told Mama he was going to do it. Mama told him to talk like he had some sense." She took a deep breath. "Tucker put his gun to his head and shot himself."

"I'm sorry to have to tell you, but in spite of all that the rescue squad, and nurses, and doctors could do, we couldn't save him."

She stared at my face, without reacting.

Until you use the word "dead" or "died," some families cling to the hope that the void looming into their lives isn't really there. Until you say "dead," their daughter, son, husband, wife, lover, friend *may* still be alive.

"We did our best," I said, "but he died."

She raised her shoulders in a gentle shrug. "Tucker's been talking about this for the last few years. He drinks. His liver's gone, his pancreas's gone, his kidneys are going, he hasn't worked in years." She shook her head. "He just stays around Mama's house, drinks, and talks about killing himself. Mama's torn up about it, but we figured it would happen sooner or later. I just hate that he did it in front of her." She gestured toward the floor. "You know, right there in her kitchen."

We stared at the floor.

I couldn't think of anything to say that would help her. Sometimes sitting quietly seems the most respectful thing to do. I waited several minutes and then gestured toward Beth. "Beth will help with the arrangements: telephone, funeral home, friends, and family. Do you want to see his body?" I kept my voice gentle, and matter-of-fact. "Some people do, and some people don't. Either way is okay."

The sister shook her head. "I already saw it at home."

I glanced over at Beth. She raised her eyebrows, but didn't speak.

I looked back at Tucker's sister. "Is there anything we can do for you?"

"Call any funeral parlor you want." She stood. "I gave my name and phone number to the lady at the desk. Is there anything else I need to sign?"

"Not that I know of." I stood, too.

"Okay." She turned and walked out the door.

Beth and I looked at each other.

"Damn." I sat back down. "That was easier than I expected."

"No shit." She shook her head and frowned. "She in denial?"

"Either that, or the guy had been such a problem for so long that he finally wore her out." Alcoholism, organ failure, suicide threats—those things get tiresome after fifteen minutes in the ER. I couldn't imagine dealing with them at home, day after day. Although Beth and I had been prepared to be with Tucker's sister through her first moments of pain, I was relieved when she walked out so abruptly. I wouldn't have to sit in a room full of his family, wouldn't have to watch them make helpless little gestures with their hands, begin to ask a question, and then murmur to a stop.

After someone's been murdered in gang violence, the family's angry. Angry at the killer, at the nurses and doctors who didn't bring him back to life, angry at everyone. The room buzzes with rage. With a suicide, the family's usually quiet, subdued, tentative.

That night, I was grateful that Tucker's sister had taken it so calmly, and had left so quietly. I'd been spared a portion of pain. Of course, she hadn't been spared anything. Neither had their mother. Suicide is an aggressive act; it unleashes a burden of guilt on everyone who survives. Many of us can imagine a life so painful and hopeless that suicide seems the least painful option, and up to a third of us will consider it at least once during our lifetime. But to do it in front of one's mom? That seemed too hostile to consider.

Perhaps those of us who somehow get through the dark moments, and stay to take the risks of living, instinctively resent those who bail out, leaving us to comfort their widows and sit down to face their sisters' empty faces. I was angry at Tucker because I felt like I'd failed him, mucking about in his blood and brains trying to stick a plastic tube down into his lungs.

I resented him for leaving such a mess, and I disliked myself for resenting him; it seemed like Tucker had enough going against him without my antipathy. Suicides are often an attempt to escape an excruciating psychic pain, from which no relief can be found. Psychiatrists have developed a test to measure hopelessness, a trait that predicts 91–94 percent of suicides. Many of those who kill themselves can literally see no other solution. A man who survived jumping from the Golden Gate Bridge said, "I still see my hands coming off the railing . . . I instantly realized that everything in my life that I'd thought was unfixable was totally fixable—except for having just jumped."

Part of the deal about being an ER doctor is that you often have to care more about people than they do themselves. Like the teenage girl with a tube snaking through her nose and down into her stomach so the nurses can squirt charcoal slurry down to absorb the poison she's taken. Black smears of powdered charcoal stain her gown, the sheets, the floor—it seems to go everywhere. Or the guy who swallows an entire bottle of Tylenol. Or the woman who slashes her wrists; or the guy who takes all his antidepressants and sits in the car while it runs. Patients are in pain, and I care about them. If I don't, I fake it until I find something that humanizes them.

As a doctor in an ER, I'm expected to at least try to resuscitate the person who's shot himself. The failure to do so carries a moral and emotional burden even when the effort seems futile from the start. I've wondered about the study my professor told us about in medical school—the one in which the traffic cops were found to be kinder than ER docs. Maybe the cops *were* more compassionate than the docs; or maybe it's harder to be emotionally open when you feel that it's somehow your fault that someone has died.

Beth and one of the other nurses washed Tucker's body, wrapped it in a sheet, and zipped it into a plastic bag. A nursing assistant rolled him down to the morgue. The ward clerk asked Carlos, from housekeeping, to mop the floor. The smears of Tucker's blood were a biohazard, a potential broth of AIDS and hepatitis that had to be cleaned up. Walking backward, Carlos swabbed the floor, the mop fanning out smoothly, side to side. When he was done, the floor had a subtle sheen: ready for the next damaged person the paramedics would bring us.

I didn't know who would clean the kitchen floor in Tucker's house. Probably his sister, maybe his mother. Would she scrub every inch of her kitchen floor, trying to expunge all traces of the shock and pain she'd been left with? Or perhaps she would hesitate, as if a spotless kitchen floor would be a betrayal, an erasure of Tucker's existence, as if she'd discarded his birth certificate, or a grade school picture, or a locket of hair she'd saved from his first haircut.

LONGING FOR SLEEP

When I finished my residency training in Pittsburgh, we moved back to North Carolina, where I spent two years as an assistant professor in the Department of Emergency Medicine at one of the medical schools. I enjoyed thinking of myself as a mentor and teacher, and had a secret hope of becoming a favorite of the house staff. I projected the persona of an enthusiastic, tenure-track academic, and within two years I had presented original research at national meetings and had published a chapter in *Rosen's*, the major textbook of our specialty. I won the Teacher of the Year Award my first year on the job. But I didn't really enjoy my accomplishments and I was exhausted from working rotating shifts, giving lectures, and writing research papers. Between clinical shifts and academic work, I could go a month without having a single day in which I didn't go into the hospital. Although I loved the idea of being an academic emergency physician, the reality of it gave me very little pleasure.

Obsessed with a career that I wasn't enjoying, I resented the fact that Sally, who had chosen to be a full-time mom, seemed to be having a great time. Sally's master's degree and nursing experience had been in adolescent psychiatry, and she believed that children can benefit from having a mother at home to nurture the development of their characters and personalities. Sally was attuned to the issues facing working mothers and stay-at-home mothers, and wished that she had the energy to do both. But she was afraid she'd feel torn if she had to call out from work because a child was sick at home. She'd rather feel calm while doing one job than tense while doing two.

Although my job paid enough for Sally to stay at home, it didn't leave me much energy to help take care of kids. With the addition of Sam, our third child, Sally was even busier than before. But she was strong, and smart, and loving, and she was doing great at her job while I hated mine.

She's since told me that many mornings after I'd pulled out of the driveway to go to the hospital, leaving her with our five-year-old, two-year-old, and newborn, she'd lean against the wall and slide down until she was sitting on the floor. Crying about the tension I'd left in my wake as I walked out of the house.

I remained relentlessly focused on making full professor, and Sally maintained her own facade of happiness, but we finally realized just how miserable we were. We decided I needed a situation where I could work my shifts and go home. With a job, rather than a career, maybe I'd relax, and feel free to take some time off. Read more, do some woodworking, spend time with the kids. A move to Durham would make us all happier.

I took four days off work so we could look for a new house. The realtor had shown us a dozen places, but there seemed to be something unsuitable about each of them. At the end of the fourth day, she showed us a house that had just come on the market. We stood at the curb, looking down a slate walkway that ran between two magnolia trees shading the front of a two-story brick house.

"I like it," Sally said, hugging my arm. We were both excited about the move.

I put my hand over Sally's, and squeezed it. I liked the dense, towering magnolias in the front yard. I liked the granite curbstone. This house, with the small brick house next door, and the white bungalow across the street, seemed perfect.

"The extra lot goes with it," the realtor told us as she led us inside. "You could probably take the woodstove insert out," she said, gesturing to the black iron doors covering the fireplace. "Nice cabinetry on either side of the fireplace."

"Oak floors," Sally said, looking at me.

"Tall ceilings, too."

Sally scrunched her shoulders and smiled. "It's nice," she whispered.

"It is, isn't it?" We wandered upstairs, down into the basement, and back outside. A car drove by and slowed down, the man and woman inside craning their necks to look at the house.

"Let's buy it," I said.

"But there isn't any place for you to sleep when you're working the night shift."

"I'll be fine." I could sleep in the basement if it came to that.

"You're just ready to buy something, it doesn't matter what," the realtor said.

Sally rolled her eyes. "You have no idea."

But what was there to discuss? It was an ideal house: safe neighborhood, shady streets, a nice mix of older houses. Even came with an extra lot. If there wasn't a quiet place for me to sleep when I was on night shift, I'd deal with it.

On the drive back, I told Sally, "I love the staircase, with the banister that curves out at the bottom."

"That was the house in Trinity Park," she said.

"Oh."

We drove through the flat green fields of Piedmont North Carolina.

"It'll be nice to have a full basement, with a workshop," I said.

"That was a different house," Sally said apologetically. "But ours has a half-basement."

"Oh." I kept driving. "Does it have a big front porch?"

"Yes," Sally said, laughing. "The porch goes all the way across."

"I really like the porch," I said, wanting to like something about the house we'd just made an offer on. "Does it have a swing?"

"Yes."

"Good, 'cause I liked it a lot."

We loved our new house, but it offered no space in which to get away from each other. That became a problem when I had to work three or four nights in a row. It's difficult to express what a grind the night shift can be. I remember pulling "all-nighters" as an undergraduate—endless cups of coffee fueled the midnight scramble to cram in enough information to pass the next morning's exam. There were runs to all-night pancake shops and small thrills of pleasure at being awake while everyone else was asleep.

The first few nights in the ER, I felt a similar frisson of excitement—but it was accompanied by crampy abdominal pain from the fear that someone would come crashing in with a problem I wouldn't be able to handle. I've talked with other ER docs, and they experienced the same gastrointestinal response to the night shifts when they first started out. Of course, no job remains an adventure forever—the night shift eventually loses its novelty, and all you want to do is get home and go to bed. But daytime sleep is fitful at best, and when it's repeatedly disrupted, it's a jangling, maddening experience.

One Saturday morning a few years after we'd moved, I came home after a busy Friday night. Chart after chart, problem after problem; I finally made it through the shift, got home, and crawled into bed.

I'd begun drifting toward sleep when Sarah started singing in her room, right next door to ours. I knew she was sitting cross-legged on her bed, earphones on. Her voice was loud and tuneless as she sang along with "Doe, a deer," from *The Sound of Music*, a video she'd seen so many times she'd memorized every line. She was almost yelling out the words. I tried to ignore her, but my head began to throb. I got up and knocked on her door. Hearing a muffled reply, I walked in.

"What?" she demanded, glaring at me. As well as having Down syndrome, Sarah was a twelve-year-old and had become as sullen and impatient as any other preteen.

"Your music." I gestured toward her earphones. "It must be up too high, because you're singing way too loud."

"No I'm not," she said, in the loud flat voice of someone who can't hear themselves.

"Take it off," I said.

"Why?" she asked, as she pulled the earpieces down to her cheeks.

"You're singing way too loud," I said. I pointed to the wall between our rooms. "I'm trying to sleep."

"Nuh uh," she said.

"If you don't sing softer, I'll take your CD player away."

"Can you just go now?"

I raised my eyebrows to let her know I meant business.

She turned the little volume knob down a fraction. "Just go," she said. "Okay?"

I turned, and went back to bed. I could barely hear her singing through the wall. Glad for the near quiet, I began to drift off. I shifted my shoulders, scrunched the pillow under my head. As my breathing slowed, I heard Sam say, "John, I didn't lose it." Sam was seven at the time, John nine.

Hopefully, Sally would intervene and I could continue drifting toward sleep.

John said something I couldn't make out through the wall.

"Johhhn," Sam said louder. "I mean it."

"You were the last one to play with it," John said, his voice scaling upwards.

I was fully awake. And I still had two more nights to go. Why wouldn't they let me sleep?

I got up, used the bathroom, and knocked on the boys' door as I walked into their room. Sam and John were facing each other. John clutched a plastic action figure.

"What's the problem?" I asked.

"Sam lost the light saber." John pointed to the empty, upraised fist of his toy.

"Did not."

I'd just finished nine hours of unrelenting problems. And I needed to sleep. I went to the hall. "Sally," I called loudly down the stairs.

She walked to the bottom of the stairs and looked up at me.

"Can you keep the boys quiet," I asked, "so I can sleep?"

"They didn't seem that loud to me," she said.

We'd been through this over and over. She had a "Princess and the Pea" theory about me and sleep. To hear her tell it, a cat walking outside would wake me. Her assertion was that I took things too personally.

But it seemed obvious to me that the need to sleep isn't personal. It's physiological. Like needing food or water or air.

Sally looked at her feet, then back up the stairs at me. "Buddy," she said, "I don't know what to tell you." She thought it was my responsibility to take care of myself.

"You don't know what to tell me?" I took a deep breath. "You could tell me you're going to do something to keep the kids quiet."

"They're kids." Sally put her arms out to the sides, palms forward. "They're going to fuss a little. That's what kids do."

I was stuck. I had to sleep. If I didn't sleep, I'd make careless mistakes at work that would hurt people. I walked back to the bedroom and stared at the clock—9:10. If I could get to sleep by 9:30, and sleep till 12:30, that would be three hours. Then I could eat lunch, sleep another three or four hours, and I'd be okay.

I put a CD of ocean sounds on, and turned up the volume. I crawled into bed, and pulled a pillow over my head. If they knew how much I needed to sleep, they'd be more thoughtful. I tried to forget about all that and concentrate on the sound of the ocean. I imagined lying on a beach, the sun beating down on me, my muscles relaxing against the hot summer sand.

I felt I was in that delicate threshold, floating up toward sleep. I imagined my brain cells settling, the chatter from ridge to ridge in the cortex dampening down. The tiny flashes of light twinkled off, like the lights in the windows of a small town, one by one, turning off, until the town is quiet and dark. The light, lazy, drifting awareness that I was slipping into sleep.

"*John!*" another plaintive yelp from Sam ricocheted into our room, jolting me awake. I jerked free from the covers, swung my legs out of bed, and put my bare feet against the cold wooden floor of the bedroom. "I can't do this. I can't keep working without sleep." There are plenty of things I don't want to do, but this was a different issue. It wasn't that I didn't *want* to keep working night shifts while my family woke me up during the day—I wasn't *able* to do it. I walked downstairs to the laundry room, where Sally was sorting laundry. "Sally," I said. "I can't do this."

She looked at me with a bored expression, then tossed a pair of jeans onto a pile of dark clothes. We'd had the argument before. She thought it was just another example of my wanting to control other people. I thought she was being passive-aggressive.

I pointed upstairs, toward the boys' room. "I don't know what I can say to make you see. I can't do it."

"Paul," Sally said, picking up one of Sarah's blouses, "I know you're exhausted, but the boys aren't making that much noise. If you hear *any* noise, you wake up." She shook her head the same way she had every other time we'd had the same argument. "And you're taking it way too personally. The boys didn't mean to wake you up." She tossed the blouse on top of the pile of whites. "They're just kids. And kids make a little noise when they play."

"I know that." I was angry that she was patronizing me. "Sally, you just don't get it. It isn't personal. It's a physiologic imperative. I've got to get to sleep."

"Physiologic imperative," Sally repeated.

"I can't do this," I said, beginning to cry. My chest began to ache. At forty-four, was I having a heart attack? If so, I wouldn't have to get to sleep, wouldn't have to go back to the ER. But I didn't get short of breath, didn't break out in a sweat, didn't have any pain in my arm, jaw, or neck. It wasn't a heart attack. I was still on the hook. "Sally," I whispered "I've got to sleep." Maybe she would see.

"Paul, I don't know what to tell you."

"Tell me you'll keep the kids quiet."

"I'm not the sleep police," she said.

"The fucking sleep police?" I raised my voice.

"You're being irrational," Sally said calmly, as she left the laundry room.

"Irrational?" I yelled, following her. "*Irrational?* I'll tell you what's irrational."

She continued walking.

"You're out of your fucking mind if you think I'm going to keep working my ass off while you and the kids wake me up every fifteen seconds. That's what's fucking irrational! If I go to work sleepy, I'll fuck up and kill somebody. You know that." I jabbed my finger toward her back. "You know it and you don't care."

Sally turned and went to the kitchen.

"I'm not going to keep doing this," I shouted. If I went nuts, maybe Sally would see how badly I needed to sleep.

"I'm not going to talk to you when you're like this," she said, as she turned to walk back to the living room.

"Not going to talk to me when I'm like this?" I could feel my voice getting hoarse, but I couldn't stop myself. "You'd *better* talk to me, because I'm not going to keep going through this every time I work a cycle of nights." It felt good to be scorching toward a resolution. Something was going to change.

As I yelled, Sally took the kids outside, onto the front porch. Was it because she knew I wouldn't hurt anyone in public?

Sally sat down in the porch swing, John on one side, Sarah on the other. Sam sat in a wicker chair.

"I can't do it," I whispered to Sally. "I just can't."

When Sam saw me crying, he thought I was joking, and laughed.

I grabbed him by the upper arms and jerked him to his feet. "I will *hurt* you," I said, through clenched teeth.

"Paul," Sally said, in a stern voice. "Give Sam to me."

"You're *telling* me?" I shook Sam hard, once, snapping his head back.

"No," her voice softened. "I'm asking."

I looked over at her.

"Please," she said gently. "Paul," she said, as if calling me from a distance. "You don't want to hurt Sam."

I looked at Sam. His face was pale, his eyes frozen wide.

"Please, Paul," Sally's voice was calm and gentle. "You don't want to hurt him."

Sally was *right*. I didn't want to hurt Sam. I looked around. The morning sun was bright. John sat pale and motionless, his mother's arm around his shoulders. He watched me like he would a snake, afraid to move. Sarah sat quietly on the other side of Sally. I wondered how much of this she understood. I looked back into Sam's face, and let go of his arms. "I'm sorry, Sam." I reached out to stroke his hair, but he pulled away. "I'm sorry," I whispered again. I walked inside, and up the stairs.

The house was empty.

The quiet was absolute.

In bed, I curled up alone.

I couldn't sleep.

SEEKING REHAB

LIKE all families, ours has had occasional meltdowns. But this one was different—for that one brief instant I'd come dangerously close to hurting Sam. It scared me. As an ER doc I'd been trained to recognize the patterns of non-accidental injuries, and to assess the family dynamics for the risk of child abuse. The presence of a child with special needs puts a family at risk. Stressful employment and rotating shifts puts a family at risk. A recent move to a new area without a broad support system puts a family at risk. I could recognize all these things in my own family, and although part of me doubted that I'd ever intentionally hurt my family, I'd come closer than I'd ever thought I would.

I wanted to blame my job for my outburst, but I couldn't. The docs I worked with often seemed frazzled, mad, and frustrated at work, but I couldn't imagine any of them chasing their family onto the front porch, or shaking a child in anger.

A few days later, Sally and I talked about it. She still wanted me to get therapy, but the solution seemed simpler to me: all I needed was sleep.

"I know you have to get your sleep," she said. "And when you're rested, you do a lot better." She leaned forward and touched my forearm. "But Paul, you seem so miserable. I can't remember the last time you were really happy."

"We're not talking about my happiness," I said. "We're talking about me getting enough sleep to do my job." It seemed axiomatic to me. I wasn't the guy who needed help—I was the guy who fixed things.

"Okay." She leaned back. "Okay."

We found a workable distance in which we could share the same bed, work together raising the kids, and avoid any conflicts that could accelerate. We maintained our routines—when I was on a daytime schedule we'd sit together in bed in the morning, sipping coffee. At night we'd prop up against the headboard to read before going to sleep. We told each other little things that happened during our day.

We remained respectful and calm, and tiptoed around the subject of my sleep as circumspectly as I wished the kids would tiptoe when I was sleeping during the day. If not intimacy, at least it wasn't acrimony. Every once in a while Sally would mention how helpful therapy had been for her, and I'd nod.

I was working at the hospital late one Saturday night or early Sunday morning. Phones rang unanswered. The paramedics' radio continued non-stop with reports of patients on the way. An old woman stood at the desk of the nurses' station, trying to catch someone's attention. A child in room 1 cried incessantly; the warning bells on the monitor in room 2 chimed unnoticed. Two paramedic units stood in the hallway next to their patients on stretchers. The "To Be Seen" rack was stuffed with charts.

I took a deep breath and picked up the next chart. Mr. Smith, a forty-five-year-old alcoholic, wanted rehabilitation. Depending on the situation, a patient "seeking rehab" can be a real-time sink.

I grabbed the next chart, a guy who'd twisted his ankle. I'd start with him, get the ankle film ordered, then go see the rehab patient. Carrying both charts, I saw the ankle, ordered the film, then went to see the alcoholic.

Mr. Smith was in room 25, a large room with a heavy sliding glass door. It's usually reserved for patients with chest pain or other problems that require monitoring. I knocked on the door, then slid it open. Mr. Smith reclined on the stretcher, the head of the stretcher raised like a chaise longue. He was a large man and sat with his arms crossed, muscular and tanned. He looked like he worked outdoors. He stared balefully from under bushy dark eyebrows. When he was sober, he was probably handsome, in spite of his coarse features. He looked like a man you'd see in magazine ads, a cowboy sitting next to a campfire, sipping coffee from a tin cup, or a construction worker, holding a cigarette between his fingers while he studied plans, the steel skeleton of a large building in the background. His hair was curly and moderately long. His fingers were thick, heavy, meaty.

In the corner, his wife sat on a plastic chair, next to a waste can and the suction equipment. A petite woman, she stood and smiled when I entered the room. Her lipstick looked freshly applied.

Mr. Smith swung his stare from me, to his wife, and back to me.

I walked to his stretcher and held out my hand.

He stared at it, then shook it. "Doc."

His wife smiled nervously.

"The triage note says you want to go to rehab."

He nodded, his eyes on mine.

"How much have you been drinking?"

"Couple of six-packs a day."

"Or more," his wife said quietly.

He swung his head to stare at her, and shrugged.

"When was the last time you were in rehab?"

"Couple of months ago." He grinned. "Walked out of that place, caught a bus to a bar, been drunk ever since."

His wife shook her head, still looking at the floor.

I made a note on the chart. "The triage note says you've had thoughts of hurting yourself."

To find him a rehab spot, I'd have to talk with someone on the phone. They'd ask me if Mr. Smith was suicidal. If he was, he'd go to Maple Lawn, a local rehab center. If there wasn't a bed available there, he'd have to go somewhere else.

He nodded again, slowly, judiciously, still maintaining good eye contact. I felt like we were playing poker, and he was raising me one. You never know if someone's really suicidal, or just knows how to play the system. Claiming to be suicidal is one way to make certain you'll get into rehab, somewhere.

"Do you have any specific plans?" Another question I'd be asked, as I tried to find him a spot.

"Yeah." He snorted. "I specifically plan to kill myself." His speech was slow, and careful, as if not to slur his words.

"How?"

"I specifically plan to drive my car into a bridge support."

"Any thoughts of hurting anyone else?"

"Not yet." His eyes bored into mine.

"He doesn't want to hurt anyone." His wife stepped forward

half a step. "He's just asking for help. You gotta understand, it was hard for him to come in tonight."

I'm an ER doctor: If you come through the doors of my department, I'll take care of you, regardless of ability or inclination to pay. I was raised in a Quaker family with a strong social conscience, and I'm proud of the fact that ER doctors don't turn anyone away. There's also a federal law requiring me to provide at least a "screening exam." The law was enacted in response to some ERs in small, private hospitals turning pregnant women away because they didn't have insurance, even though they were in active labor.

It's shameful such a law is necessary. The law requires emergency physicians to determine if a true emergency exists. Of course, once you do a screening exam, you may as well complete the exam and render treatment. It only takes a few more minutes, and most people would go ballistic if we denied them treatment.

ER doctors treat anybody, any time, for any problem, regardless of ability to pay. At my hospital, we don't even have the insurance information on the chart when we see the patient. I like it that way: If you have chest pain, don't worry. We'll get you taken care of. Kid have an earache? Glad to help.

Unless you want rehabilitation for alcohol or other drugs. The state of North Carolina doesn't provide free rehab for alcohol or drug addiction. Neither does the federal government. And it's obviously not a service the ER can provide. If you have insurance that covers substance abuse, you can go into a private rehab center. If not, you go home and follow up with the Durham County Substance Abuse Services the next morning. The only exception is if you're suicidal: then you'll get a bed somewhere. Durham County has contracted for a limited number of beds in the local private rehab center, and they'll allot a bed to a county resident who's suicidal and needs rehab. If those beds are full, you go to a state hospital.

If I had my way, we'd just total up the costs: rehab, trauma, and medical care. Then tax alcohol sales accordingly. Let the cost of a six-pack or a bottle of wine reflect the true cost to society. Use the money to pay for rehab. But I don't have my way. I'm just the guy who has to ask an alcoholic or a crack addict if he has insurance.

I looked from Mr. Smith, to his wife, and then back to him. "I'm an ER doctor. I'm glad to take care of you whether you have insurance or not." I took a breath. "But. I'm going to make a call, to try to find you a rehab bed. If you have insurance, I call one guy. If you don't have insurance, I call a different guy."

"I've got insurance." His wife sat, put her pocketbook on her lap, and scrambled through it.

"Is his name on your policy?"

"No," she looked up. "But I can put his name on it Monday."

"Like I said, I'm glad to take care of him, regardless. But if his name isn't on the policy now, they won't take it. I'll call the Durham County crisis worker, do my best to get him in."

"Please." She smiled, and tilted her head to the side. *Be a sport. Get my husband into rehab.*

I paged the crisis worker on call for Durham County Mental Health, and checked on the other patient's ankle film. There was a tiny fleck of bone that had been pulled loose from the lateral malleolus. I asked a physician's assistant to put him in a splint, and finished with the chart.

The next chart in the rack was a three-year-old child with a fever. Maybe I could knock that out while I waited for Mental Health to call back. The girl was sitting in her mother's lap watching me with unwavering eyes as I walked into the room. The mother, somewhere in her twenties, had dark skin; she was wearing a puffy pink jacket and faded blue jeans. She was frowning—must've been waiting a while. The infant was wearing a child's hospital gown, open at the back.

Another girl, who looked to be about five years old, sat in a plastic chair next to the stretcher. She was swinging her feet, and wore black patent leather shoes and white socks.

I looked at the name on the chart. K'isha. Not sure how to pronounce it, I looked at the mother. "Keesha?"

"*Ka*-isha." Her tone had a brittle edge.

"Ka-isha," I repeated. "It's a pretty name." I looked over at K'isha and smiled.

She scrunched her face into a scowl and turned it into her mother's chest.

"How long has she been having a fever?"

"Two days."

After the questions about cough, nausea, vomiting, and diarrhea, it was time to examine K'isha. I'd already noted that she wasn't lethargic and wasn't having problems breathing. She had good muscle tone and was responding normally to her environment. So far, she hadn't started crying, but she looked scared. You can listen to the lung sounds of a crying child gasping for air, but it's easier to get a good exam if they're not howling. It's worth it to take a few minutes.

I pulled the stethoscope from around my neck, and turned toward the five-year-old sister. "What's your name?"

"Latoya."

K'isha twisted in her mother's lap to look at her sister.

"I'm going to listen to *Latoya's* breathing." I spoke with the same gentle cadence I'd used when reading *Pat the Bunny* to my children when they were small enough to snuggle next to me on the couch. I put the stethoscope into my ears, and leaned down to place the stethoscope on Latoya's chest.

Latoya grinned up at her mother.

I listened to the five-year-old's chest for a moment, then pulled the stethoscope from my ears. "You don't smoke, do you?"

She shook her head solemnly.

"I could tell, because your lungs sound so healthy." Placing my stethoscope back into my ears, I turned to the mother. "Now I'm going to listen to *Mommy's* chest." K'isha glared at my hand as I placed the stethoscope over her mother's heart, but she didn't pull away.

"Now I'm going to listen to *Latoya* again."

Latoya pulled her shoulders back, and pushed her chest out. She grinned, enjoying what was clearly a game.

"Now I'm going to listen to *Mommy* again."

The mother smiled for the first time.

After I listened to the mother's chest, I pulled back. "Do you want me to listen to *your* chest?"

K'isha didn't move. I gently placed the stethoscope against her back, to listen to the posterior lung fields. She hunched her shoulders and clung tighter to her mother, but didn't cry. I moved the stethoscope across each lung field. They were all clear—the fever wasn't from pneumonia.

I pulled the otoscope from the bracket on the wall. "I'm going to look in *Latoya's* ears."

She tilted her head, offering her left ear.

"Latoya's got *pretty* ears," I said, as I pretended to look in the left, then right ear. I turned toward the mother. "Now I'm going to look in *Mommy's* ears."

The mother smiled again, wide enough to show dimples on both cheeks.

K'isha watched with interest. "You want to look in Mommy's ears?"

K'isha leaned over to look through the otoscope, her curiosity overcoming her mistrust.

"Let me look." Latoya stood on her tiptoes. "Move, K'isha."

"Careful," I said.

K'isha pulled her head back, and Latoya peered through the otoscope.

"Now I'm going to look in *K'isha's* ears."

"Let me see first." Latoya tugged at my scrub pants.

"Latoya, sit down," the mother said.

K'isha's right eardrum was normal—a delicate, translucent oval membrane at the end of the external canal. Her left eardrum bulged out—ugly, red, and inflamed.

"She's got an ear infection," I told her mother, as I hung the otoscope back in its holder. "I'll write a prescription for azithromycin. She'll need to take it for five days. We'll give her the first dose here."

"I thought it might be her ears. Is it the pink medicine?"

"That's amoxicillin—you give it three times a day for ten days. What I'm suggesting is azithromycin. It's only once a day, for five days."

"You got an office somewhere?"

"No," I said, "I'm just pure ER." I appreciated her unspoken compliment, the implication that if I did have an office, she'd want me to be her children's doctor. "You've got good kids."

She tilted her head, and looked from K'isha to Latoya. "They *are* good kids." She nodded and smiled again. "Thank you."

K'isha's mother had seemed irritated at first, even before I inadvertently offended her by mispronouncing her daughter's name. I was glad I'd been able to win her over and make her smile. The first few times I played with a child during the physical exam, I just wanted to get the job done efficiently—if a child doesn't cooperate, I have to find two nurses to wrestle him down to the stretcher so I can look in the ears and throat. Finding holding help usually takes longer than the exam itself. So, spending a few minutes playing is much quicker. It's also more fun—for me, the child, and the parents.

I was writing K'isha's prescription when Maurice, one of the Mental Health crisis workers, returned his page. He's got this Jamaican accent, and sounds pleasant no matter what time of the day or night you're talking to him. I made my pitch, and gave him all of the information.

"Paul, I wish I could help you, but our beds at Maple Lawn are full. He'll have to go to Umstead."

Damn. "He's not going to like Umstead."

"I don't know what else to tell you. He's left us no choice. You can't let him go if he's suicidal."

"Yeah, I know."

"Do you think he's really suicidal"—I heard Maurice yawn over the phone—"or just working the system?"

"Don't know. But say he's bullshitting; if he died in a car wreck tonight, I'm responsible."

"Then it's Umstead," Maurice said in a calm voice. "You ready for the authorization code?"

He gave me a series of numbers I entered on the first page of a four-page form. Without an authorization code, Umstead would send Mr. Smith back. The first fifteen or so patients I sent them, I completed every blank on the form. Then I started skipping some of the blanks that seemed unnecessary. It turned out, the only line you really have to fill out is the authorization code. I wrote in the last digit.

I wished I could be as calm as Maurice.

I got the commitment papers and filled them out. Name, address, specific reasons I thought Mr. Smith needed to be committed. I filled out every line: magistrates require more information than the intake people at John Umstead. My signature had to be witnessed by a notary public. I paged the hospital nursing supervisor. They're all notaries. While I waited for her, I filled out the two-page form the federal government requires for every transfer. The first few times I transferred an uninsured suicidal patient to John Umstead, I worried I wasn't following the spirit of the law. It turns out that the law allows each state to deal with mental health however it chooses. And this is the system North Carolina has adopted. I filled out every line of that form, too. The federal people are even more detail-oriented than the magistrate.

The nursing supervisor stood behind me and watched over my shoulder as I signed the commitment paper. She stamped it with her seal and I handed it to Kevin, the charge nurse. "Let's put Mr. Smith into seclusion, until the sheriff's department gets here." The deputies transport all commitments to John Umstead. State policy again.

"Have you told him you're doing it?"

"Not yet." I put Mr. Smith's chart in the rack. "Call Security. They can go with me when I tell him."

Once, when I was an intern, I told a suicidal drunk he was being committed. He jumped off the stretcher and punched me in the side of the neck so hard it knocked me off my feet. He ran down the hall, and I scrambled up to follow him. Suzy, one of the ER nurses, yelled after me to let him go. Probably good advice, but I jumped up and chased him anyway. The patient slowed down at a door, where a security guard grabbed him. The guard and I wrestled him to the floor until other nurses and security officers got to us, and we fought him onto a stretcher. After we'd gotten leather restraints on each wrist and ankle, a nurse pointed to my shirt.

We didn't wear scrubs where I trained; we wore white coats, shirts, and ties. The women wore similarly dressy clothes. It was thought to show respect for the patients. That night, I was wearing my favorite shirt. Sally had made it of unbleached muslin. She'd used French seams, so there were no raw edges. The collar and cuffs were perfect. The arms let into the yoke without a wrinkle. It was a custom-made, perfectly tailored shirt. You couldn't buy a better shirt from a tailor in Italy, New York, anywhere in the world. And my wife had made it for me, as a gift.

The drunk had pulled out his IV when he jumped off the stretcher and as we wrestled, smeared blood all over my shirt. "I'll be back in a second." I went to the cabinet where the nurses' scrubs were stored, grabbed a top, and went to the men's bathroom. I stripped off my shirt, ran cold water into the sink, and dunked in the shirt. Peroxide's great for getting blood out of cloth, but I was afraid it would mess up the fabric. I looked in the mirror, but didn't see any blood on my skin. My neck was getting sore. *Damn.* I slipped into the green scrub top. If I left my shirt in the bathroom, someone might steal it. I went to the supply cabinet, grabbed a disposable bedpan, and went back to the bathroom. I filled it with cold water, pressed the shirt into the water, and carried it back to the nurses' station, where I slid it under a counter.

"What's this?" Suzy, the nurse who'd told me to let the man go, pointed at the bedpan.

"Sally made this shirt, and the guy in room seven got blood on it."

"She *made* it?"

"Yeah," I answered proudly.

The nurse assigned to the suicidal patient walked up. "He wants to talk with you."

I looked at my watch. I had another fifteen minutes on my shift. "What's to say? He's been committed."

"He wants to apologize." She turned to look toward the room. "It may be therapeutic."

"Therapeutic?" Suzy snorted. "He's in four-point restraints. That's all the therapy he needs."

She was probably right. But the guy'd asked to apologize. I walked to his room. "The nurse said you wanted to talk to me?"

"Yeah, sorry about all that . . . " He waved his hand in the small arc the leather restraint allowed. "You know."

I waited.

"Is there any way you could let these restraints loose?" He shrugged his right shoulder. "I mean, I'm sorry and everything, but I really don't need to be committed."

Since then, whenever I tell a patient he's being committed, I always have someone else with me.

I turned to Kevin. "If he tries to leave before Security gets here, overhead-page me. I'll help contain him 'till they show up."

While I waited for the security guards, I picked up the chart of a thirty-eight-year-old woman who was having pain whenever she urinated. *Good. That should be quick.*

Her hair was dark at the roots. She had a plain face and a timid smile. She was stocky but not obese. After she'd told me her symptoms, I did a physical exam. Her abdomen was soft, and just a little tender in the spot above the bladder. I'd just finished examining her when the overhead speaker squawked. "Dr. Austin to room twenty-five. Dr. Austin to room twenty-five."

"Excuse me," I said, and walked toward the door. "We'll check a urinalysis. I'll be back to talk with you when I get the results."

The woman said, "Okay," as I hurried out.

Two security officers stood in the hallway. Mr. Smith stood at the end of the stretcher, his arms crossed in front of his chest, glaring at them. "The fuck you want?"

"I tried to get you a spot at Maple Lawn," I said, "but they didn't have any beds."

He looked at me. "So?"

"The safe thing to do is for you to go to John Umstead."

"I'll be goddamned." He puffed his chest out.

"I've already committed you. And once someone's been committed, they wait for transportation in a seclusion room."

"Fuck all that." He pointed at me, sighting down his finger. "Somebody's gonna get hurt, you try to put me into some goddamn seclusion room."

"That'll be up to you . . . " My voice didn't shake, but I could feel my heart rate go up. "When it's all over, I'm gonna write a report." I lifted my right hand. "It may say, 'Patient stated seclusion unnecessary, but cooperated.'" I lifted my left hand. "Or it could say, 'Patient knocked out doctor's tooth, then was wrestled into seclusion.'"

He grinned.

"You knock out someone's tooth, they'll keep your ass in Umstead forever. You cooperate, who knows?" I shrugged. "Maybe you can talk your way out tonight."

He held my stare.

"Honey," his wife said, reaching out tentatively toward the man, "it may not be so bad."

He didn't move. "Shut up, bitch."

She froze.

Is this how I'd looked to Sally on our front porch? I pushed the thought away to focus on the problem at hand. We stood silently. The second hand on the clock behind the patient continued sweeping forward. I had to get the urinalysis ordered on the woman with the urinary tract infection, and there were four more charts in the rack.

"Whatever you want to do," I said, "now's the time."

"Ain't this some shit?" He raised his eyebrows as if bewildered, and turned to his wife. "Come to get some help, just trying to get some fucking *help*, and they lock your ass up like a criminal." He shook his head. "I'll go into your little room, but it's all chickenshit." He swaggered out of the room, one security guy in front and one behind him. "Pure-ass *chickenshit*!" he yelled, as he turned to walk down the hall.

The room seemed abnormally quiet without his loud hostility.

"He don't mean nothing by it," his wife said softly. She daubed under her eye with her right forefinger.

I gave the woman with the urinary tract infection a prescription for an antibiotic and a medication that would anesthetize her bladder, and make her pee bright orange. "It'll stain your underwear," I told her. "You may want to use a pad."

"Thanks." She wrinkled her nose. Then she leaned forward and whispered, "That man sure was mad."

"Saturday night in Durham."

At the end of the shift, Kevin told me that Mr. Smith raged and cursed in the seclusion room until he finally got hoarse. When the deputies arrived, he meekly walked with them to their cruiser and waited like a child at the back door of the car until one of the deputies opened it for him.

The next morning, I went home and had a cup of decaf coffee, ate a bowl of Cheerios, and stared at the wall in the kitchen. Sally sat at the table, reading the paper. The kids were upstairs, getting dressed for Sunday School.

Sally folded the paper. "So, how was your night?"

"Saturday night in the ER." I ate a spoonful of cereal. "Had a drunk who wanted rehab. Said he was suicidal. Didn't have insurance, didn't want to go to Umstead."

Sally waited.

It's hard to know how much to tell her. Even during the rough spots in our marriage, she wants to listen and offer love and support. But sometimes I get going about work and have a hard time stopping. The stories develop their own momentum and continue to pour out, even though I can see that listening takes a toll. Sometimes Sally leans back in the chair, crosses her arms, and frowns as I talk. When she catches herself sitting with a closed-off posture, she'll lean forward, uncross her arms, smile, and say, "That sounds frustrating," or some other stock phrase people in the trade use when they want to keep a nut case talking. That's when I know to shut up. I try to stick to funny stories, or little triumphs. The spinal tap on the huge, fat guy that I got with one stick. The cute kid with a chin laceration.

"The guy was hostile, threatening." I looked at Sally and sipped my coffee. "But I got him into seclusion without anyone getting hurt."

"That's good."

"Yeah, it is." I looked her in the eyes. "And it's good to be home."

Sally looked down at the newspaper, then back to me. She didn't mention the time I'd gotten knocked off my feet, or the damp shirt I brought home the next day. And she didn't mention me grabbing Sam on our front porch, or the calm she'd put in her voice when she'd asked me not to hurt him.

"I'm sorry," I said.

Sally raised her eyebrows in a question.

"For chasing you guys out onto the porch," I said. "And for grabbing Sam." I was ashamed of the fear that I'd seen in Sam's eyes, and the forced calm I'd heard in Sally's voice. I wanted her to give me absolution.

She touched my hand, then got up and walked out of the kitchen.

PART THREE

SOMEBODY'S BABY

THE rescue squad was pushing the stretcher down the hall at a near run. A firefighter rode on the side of the gurney, like a kid holding onto the side of a grocery cart. He leaned over the patient's chest, and counted loudly, "One-one thousand, two-one thousand, three-one thousand," each time he pumped on the patient's rib cage. A paramedic scrambled at the head of the stretcher, her black boots dancing sideways, a quick criss-cross, right-left-right. Her hands were busy, too—with her right hand she held a mask against the patient's face, and with her left she squeezed a bag, forcing air into the lungs. Both gloves were smeared with blood.

A woman standing at the desk of the nurses' station pulled her little boy to her. They both stared with their mouths open as the knot of people hurried past.

I leaned over to the unit secretary. "Page the trauma team."

"Just did."

I went to the room designated for trauma cases. Someone had turned on the suction line. Its hissing was barely audible above the bustle of people preparing to move the patient to our stretcher.

"There's one more strap." Barry, the chief paramedic, pointed to the end of the stretcher. "At her feet."

A firefighter squeezed the black plastic clasp, and flicked the orange webbing free. "Okay."

Barry grasped the yellow plastic backboard. Lisa, the ER nurse, leaned over our stretcher to help. She grabbed one of the handholds and in a swift arc they whisked the patient over to our stretcher. "Twelve-year-old, hit by a car," Barry continued. "I tried to intubate her with a 6-0 tube but it wouldn't go in. Vocal cords were too small." He winced. "Tried again with a pediatric tube, but couldn't see the cords the second time." He handed an IV bag to Lisa. She stretched up on her toes to secure the bag to the hook suspended from the ceiling. Barry wiped his forehead on his shirtsleeve. "We were right around the corner, so we decided to scoop and run. She had a pulse at the scene. Lost it en route."

The firefighter who'd been doing compressions on the girl's chest glanced around the floor. "Is there a stool anywhere?" He stood on his toes and started doing compressions again. He needed to be higher, to be centered over her chest. Someone left, presumably to find a stool. The paramedic at the head fitted the face mask against the girl's chin and nose, then began squeezing the green football-shaped bag again, pumping oxygen into her lungs.

I grabbed a pair of exam gloves and slipped through the people crowded around the stretcher.

The left side of the girl's face had been torn to a ragged red pulp, and a small, bloody tag was all that remained of her left ear. A cervical collar kept her neck rigid, but her head jostled with every compression of her chest.

If someone comes in pulseless after blunt trauma, it's unlikely you'll be able to resuscitate them. But when it's a kid, you want to work a code as long as you can. It's human nature. And the first step, without which all others are futile, is to secure the airway. In every advanced life support class you learn "A" is for Airway; "B" is for Breathing; and "C" is for Circulation. Until you secure the airway, all other efforts are useless. All the fancy doctoring in the world can't keep someone alive without an airway.

As I reached for the laryngoscope and a tube, Barry tapped me on the shoulder. "You better go with a 4-0 tube. I couldn't get a 6-0 in."

Barry had been a paramedic longer than I'd been a doctor. I hesitated. Just looking at the girl, a 6-0 looked more like the right size. But if he'd tried one, and it wouldn't go . . . I looked at Barry. "You got a good look at the cords?"

"I was staring right at them. That's what was so frustrating. The 6-0 was just too damn big." He shook his head.

I clicked the lighted blade onto the laryngoscope handle and picked out a 4-0 tube. "It looks small." I opened her mouth, and using the laryngoscope blade swept the tongue to the left. I advanced the laryngoscope to her epiglottis, the fleshy trap door that covers the vocal cords, and lifted it out of my way. The cords were big and white and inviting. I slipped the 4-0 tube in place.

The respiratory therapist took over. She taped the tube in place, hooked her bag to it, and squeezed.

"I'm barely ventilating her. The tube is too small."

The girl's chest hardly rose each time the bag was squeezed.

Ben Smith, a trauma surgeon, walked briskly into the room. "What do we have?"

"Kid, hit by a car," I said. "Had a pulse at the scene."

"Excuse me." Ben slipped between nurses and paramedics to stand next to the patient. "Exam gloves?"

A nurse handed him a pair of gloves. He snapped them on, and felt for the femoral pulse. "I'm getting a good pulse with compressions." He looked at the sweating firefighter doing the compressions. "Hold CPR."

The firefighter straightened up. He stretched his arms over his head, leaned backwards to stretch his back.

"No pulse." Ben looked at the paramedic. "Continue CPR."

The firefighter resumed his rhythmic pumping on the girl's chest.

Ben looked over to me and raised his eyebrows.

I shrugged.

"How old is she?" Ben glanced at her breasts and pubic hair.

"Bystanders said she was twelve."

"Then let's work this a little longer." He looked at the IV bags. "We've got her fluids wide open, right?"

"I've got a second IV here." Lisa looked up from the catheter sticking out of the girl's forearm, slowly dripping dark blood. "Gimme a line." Another nurse handed her an IV line.

"I may have to change the tube," I said to Ben. "This one's barely ventilating her."

Ben nodded to me, and turned to Lisa. "Make sure the fluids are wide open."

"They are."

Ben looked to the paramedic. "How long she been down?"

Barry glanced at his watch. "About twenty minutes."

The respiratory therapist squeezed the Ambu-bag, and frowned. "What size tube did you use?"

"A 4-0." I listened to the girl's chest with my stethoscope. First the right side, then the left. The girl's breasts were small, with dark brown nipples. "We're barely ventilating her." I looked over to Lisa. "Does she look older than twelve to you?"

"I don't know." Lisa shrugged. "Yeah, maybe."

Barry was standing behind Lisa. "The bystander said she was twelve."

Any tube is better than none at all, and with the 4-0 in place, I had some time to think. I'd had no trouble seeing the cords, and a 6-0 would've fit easily. Of course, if I took out the 4-0, and for some reason couldn't reintubate her, I was fucked. I held the tip of a 6-0 tube to her nostril. It would fit into her nostril, which is a good rule of thumb that it'll fit through the cords. "You said a 6-0 wouldn't fit?"

Barry nodded emphatically.

"The 4-0's obviously too small. I'm going to pull it and try with this one."

Barry raised his eyebrows and shook his head.

I pulled the 4-0 tube out and tossed it on the floor, clicked the blade into the laryngoscope, and peered down her throat. I could see the epiglottis, but not the cords. "Gimme some cricoid pressure."

The respiratory therapist pushed down gently on the front of the girl's neck, forcing her windpipe further into my field of vision.

"I still don't see the cords." I pulled up harder on my laryngoscope. "Can you give me more cricoid?"

"I'm pushing as hard as I can."

I still couldn't see the cords. I pulled the laryngoscope out. "Bag her up some, lemme change blades."

The respiratory therapist scrambled to put the face mask

back on the bag. "Can someone hold the mask against the face for me?"

Lisa gripped the girl's jaw with her fingers, and pressed the mask against the bloody face with her thumbs.

"Thanks." The respiratory therapist squeezed the bag, inflating the girl's chest, which rose and fell steadily. We were ventilating her better with the mask than we had with the 4-0 tube.

I changed over to a curved blade, and checked the bulb. It worked. "Okay." I gestured to the respiratory therapist, and she pulled the bloody mask out of my way.

I swept the tongue to the left, saw the epiglottis, but still couldn't see the cords. "*Damn.*" I pulled up harder. "Gimme some cricoid." The epiglottis stubbornly covered the cords. I should've left the 4-0 in place. Been satisfied with what I had. "Bag her up some more. I'm going back to the straight blade." Why couldn't I see the cords? The first time I tubed her, the cords were as big and wide as a door at the end of a hall.

"You can't get the airway?" Ben moved toward the head of the stretcher.

"Yeah," I said, "I'll get it." I clicked the straight blade back into the laryngoscope. *Please, let me get it.* Why did I pull the first tube out? I wiped the sweat from my forehead on the sleeve of my scrub tops. Just *had* to change the tube, didn't I?

I looked again, but couldn't see the cords. Time slowed down as in a nightmare. Where were the fucking cords? I straightened up. "Bag her up again."

The respiratory therapist pumped air into the girl with the face mask.

"Gimme a scalpel," Ben said. He wanted to cut a hole in her neck to stick in a tube.

The chatter in the room stopped, and everyone stared at me.

"Goddamn, Ben. I'll get it." I motioned the therapist to remove the mask. *Please*. I got the tongue to the side, and the cords popped into view like a huge billboard. "Gimme the tube." The therapist placed the 6-0 tube in my hand. I eased it down between the cords with plenty of room. "It's in." I straightened, and took a deep breath. *Thank you thank you thank you.*

The respiratory therapist hooked the bag to the tube, and squeezed. The girl's chest expanded briskly and fully. "That's better."

"How much fluid has she had?" With Airway and Breathing back where they should be, Ben had moved to Circulation again.

"This'll be her third liter."

"Pulseless after blunt trauma . . ." Ben didn't finish his sentence. Everyone in the room knew this was a dead girl: we just hadn't admitted it yet. I took a deep breath and let it out slowly. At least now she was a dead girl with the right-sized endotracheal tube: I'd done all I could do.

We stared at the girl as Barry pumped on her chest and the respiratory therapist pumped air into her lungs.

"Hold CPR." Ben kept his fingers on the femoral pulse. "Nothing. Continue CPR." He looked over at me. "Paul, unless you have any ideas . . ."

Studies have shown that people who are pulseless after blunt trauma are dead, no matter what you do. Still, it's hard to give up on a kid. "Anyone else got any ideas?"

The nurses, respiratory therapists, paramedics, and X-ray techs looked at the floor, or shrugged.

I looked around the room. "I'm ready to call it, unless anyone wants to continue."

"Time of death," Lisa called out clearly, "14:53."

I tried to smile. "Good job, team. It was a good effort. We just didn't have enough to work with."

As people drifted away from the stretcher, another paramedic walked in. "Is this the forty-year-old that was hit by a car?"

"Forty? They said she was twelve." I looked at her body. The breasts sagged limply to the sides, the pubic hair was thick and profuse and wove all the way up to her umbilicus. The left side of her face was still a ragged red mess, but the right side no longer looked like a kid's. "You sure you have the right dad with the right patient?"

"He showed up at the scene as we were leaving. Said he was her father."

"Lemme go talk with him. Where is he, the Family Room?" I stripped off my protective gear.

"Yeah."

"Do we have a name?"

"Patient's name is Crystal."

Barry, the chief paramedic, winced. "I don't know why I couldn't get the tube."

"Don't feel bad." I patted his arm. "It was a tough tube."

"Do you think she's really forty?"

"When she first got here, she looked like a big kid. Now she looks like a small woman." I washed my hands in the sink in the corner. "If the bystanders had said she was forty, she would've looked forty from the get-go." I dried my hands and tossed the paper towel into the trash.

Lisa went with me to talk with the father.

* * *

An old man sat in a chair in the corner of the Family Room—a small, windowless room, with reproductions of impressionistic art on the wall. He had a scant fringe of white hair around a shiny bald scalp, and bristly white eyebrows. He leaned forward in his chair, his knobby hands resting on the top of an aluminum cane.

I sat down in the chair next to his. "You're Crystal's father?"

He bobbed his head. His face showed no emotion.

"She was hit by a car . . ." I said softly.

His head bobbed again. "I know." He looked at his hands folded over the top of his cane. "I was there when they were leaving."

I took a deep breath. "When she got here, her heart wasn't beating."

He nodded, as if the news wasn't surprising.

"The rescue squad, nurses, and doctors did all we could."

"I know you did." He stared at his knuckles.

"And I'm sorry, but in spite of all we did, we couldn't get her heart started again." I spoke slowly, softly, clearly. "She died."

He was motionless. "She was the baby in the family," he whispered.

"I'm sorry."

He swung his large, dark brown eyes to mine. "All growed up, but still my baby girl."

We sat.

Lisa cleared her throat. "Some people want to see their loved ones, others don't."

The old man looked at Lisa.

"Would you like to see her?"

He slowly stood. "Yes, ma'am, I would."

I walked beside the old man, consciously making myself go

slowly. Patients continued to flow into the ER, and if I didn't pull their charts from the rack and go see them, the place would grind to a traffic jam that wouldn't clear till tomorrow morning. I took a deep breath. The old man deserved at least a few more minutes. We walked past patients on stretchers in the hallway. I kept my eyes on the floor to avoid making eye contact.

In the resuscitation room, a fresh sheet was tucked in around Crystal's shoulders, covering her body. Gauzes covered the raw left side of her face. Most of the blood on the floor had been hastily wiped up, but a thin smear of red remained next to the stretcher. The paper wrappers from IV catheters, gauze, endotracheal tubes had been swept up and thrown away.

The old man peered at the torn, dead face, then back to me. "I think it's her." He pulled her hand from under the sheet and stared at the long, shiny red nails. "Yeah, that's my baby," he said, as he gently laid her flaccid hand on the stretcher. He shook his head slightly, and leaned on his cane, staring at the shiny red nails against the crisp white sheet.

He reached out and touched the limp hand on the stretcher.

I stared at Crystal's body, relieved that she was forty instead of twelve. When I'd gotten to work that day, like every day, I went to my locker. There, I slipped into my running shoes, draped a stethoscope around my neck, put a pen in the pocket of my scrub shirt and trauma shears in the back pocket of my scrub bottoms. As I walked out into the emergency department, I felt the "ER Doc Paul" come forward. Curmudgeon, detached clinician, sometime jokester. A game face to help me through the shift.

When Crystal came crashing in, she was a twelve-year-old kid. Kids have a way of darting past the ER persona and staring into your naked eyes. When a child dies in the ER, or comes in dead and stays dead, the department slows down. A child's death affects all of us: nurses, doctors, ward clerks, nursing assistants. All of our masks come off. Even at forty, Crystal was too young to die. But as I stared at her dead, adult body, I felt my mask settle comfortingly back into place. I knew I could face the rest of my shift without feeling the urge to cry.

Joanne, the charge nurse, motioned to me from the hall.

I walked over.

"There's a chest pain in room two," she said. "Looks sick."

"I'll be there in a minute," I said quietly. "EKG ordered?"

She nodded.

"Thanks," I said. "Be there in a sec." I walked back into Crystal's room. "Sir, if you have any questions or concerns, call me here in the ER. They'll know how to get in touch with me."

He nodded, and limped slowly out of the room and down the hall, leaving his baby under the white sheet.

SLEEPING AT MY MOTHER-IN-LAW'S

"SAM has a birthday party he's going to this afternoon," Sally said. "John wants to invite a friend over to play."

I'd just gotten home from a night shift, dealing with every unlucky and unloved soul in Durham. *I should be exempt from further decision making.* I poured boiling water onto the decaf coffee in the single-cup filter.

"I haven't told John yes or no," Sally said.

I tossed the coffee grounds into the compost jar.

"It's been a while since he's had a friend over," Sally said.

"Who's he want to invite?"

"Lewis," she said.

Lewis was a good kid, but a little too energetic. And too loud. "As long as they stay outside, it should be okay."

"Are you sure?" Sally asked. Neither of us wanted a repeat of the scene on the front porch.

"As long as they stay outside."

"Fair enough," Sally said. "I'll get Sarah up before you get in bed."

I rinsed my bowl and cup, put them in the dishwasher, and

went upstairs. In our bedroom, I stripped off my scrubs, underwear, and socks. My underarms felt sticky. I took a quick shower, then slipped into bed.

A few minutes later, I heard Sally talking with Sarah. I couldn't make out the words, but Sally's voice was reasonable and firm. Sarah's was strident and stubborn.

I was tired of having a daughter with an extra chromosome that dulled her intellect and made her, at times, obdurately stubborn. I loved Sarah, but hated the unending daily struggles. Having a preteen around is one thing; one with Down syndrome is another.

I pulled Sally's pillow over my head.

"*No!*" Sarah yelled.

Poor Sally. Trying to get Sarah out of bed without disturbing me was a classic no-win endeavor. I had a few days off, so it wasn't mandatory that I sleep. Maybe I could just tough it out, stay up all day.

"Mom," Sarah yelled, "just leave!"

I needed to pee.

Tossing the blankets to the side, I rolled out of bed, slipped on a pair of jeans, and went to the bathroom. I looked at myself in the mirror, yawned, and sucked in my stomach. I stretched, then walked down the hall to Sarah's room. I lightly knocked on her door and cracked it open.

"Sally?"

She came to the door. "Sorry, Buddy," she said in a low voice. "Sarah's being stubborn."

"Don't worry," I said. "I think I'll get up, maybe take a nap when the kids are all out of the house."

"Thanks," Sally said.

"Sarah," I said through the crack in the door, "you want me to help you get dressed?"

"No," Sarah said loudly. "Mom can help me." In spite of her Down syndrome, Sarah had developed a high degree of modesty.

"How can Mom help you," I asked, "when you're being so stubborn?"

"I won't be stubborn," Sarah answered in a softer voice.

"Thanks." Sally winked, and closed the door.

I put on a flannel shirt, stepped into a pair of house slippers, and went downstairs to the kitchen, with its lingering smell of coffee. I sat at the table and looked at the paper. The words on the page began to blur. I crossed my arms on the table, and put my head down.

Sarah clomped into the kitchen. "Mom" she said loudly, "Sam and John ate all the Honeycomb cereal."

I jerked awake.

Sarah stood next to the trash can, clutching an empty cereal box.

I sat up and stretched. Maybe I'd go back upstairs.

"Do you want to put it on the list?" Sally asked, from the front room.

Sarah walked over to the small clipboard next to the refrigerator, and wrote something on the grocery list. It probably said, "Hony Com Cerel." If you knew what we were out of, you could make it out.

Sally walked into the kitchen. "You okay?"

"Sure." I got up and went to the half-bath. Beside the toilet there was a magazine rack, filled with out-of-date magazines and clothing catalogues that lagged a season. As I sat on the toilet, I flipped through a *New Yorker*, but I'd looked at all the cartoons so many times I knew the punch lines before I read them. I dropped it into the rack, and pulled out a magazine-sized publication, *Wellness for Emergency Physicians*.

I didn't remember sending off for it. It seemed like it had just shown up in the mail one afternoon. I'd already read the articles entitled "Using Circadian Principles in Emergency Medicine Scheduling" and "Financial Planning." They were well written, as was the one on "Health, Diet, and Exercise." An article called "Violence in the Emergency Department" was excellent. "Violence and the fear of violence is a regular concern of virtually every person who spends regular time in an emergency department," it said. It was a relief to find out that I wasn't the only one who found the ER stressful.

In another article I read that "An emergency physician often is required to manage a diverse patient population within a very short period of time." *Well, yeah.* "Some issues troubling emergency physicians can be traced to a sense of relative powerlessness." *No shit.* "Shift work is the bane of the existence of the emergency physician." *Yes*. It just felt good to hear someone else say the same things I'd been feeling. If I came home physically, emotionally, and spiritually depleted, maybe it wasn't because something was wrong with me.

I took the magazine with me back into the kitchen.

Sally was unloading the dishwasher. "Why don't you go back upstairs? It should be pretty quiet from here on out."

"I think I will." I snuggled into bed with the *Wellness* guide and opened it to the piece on "The Medical Family." I read a few lines, and felt myself fade away. I slept until lunchtime, got up, and went downstairs. Sally had the boys in the yard, picking up sticks and sweeping the walk. Sarah was swinging on the swing set.

John walked over. "How's it going, Dad?"

"Sleepy," I said. "A little grumpy, but not too bad."

"Oh."

"Mom said you were going to have Lewis over?"

"If it's okay."

"Sure," I said. "But can you guys stay outside?"

"Oh, yeah," John said. "Don't worry about that."

"You're going to a birthday party?" I called out to Sam.

"Yeah," he said, bending over to pick up another stick. "It's gonna be great."

I walked inside, and ate some pre-washed carrots and a cup of yogurt. I started reading the piece on "The Medical Family" again. There was a section on "Perils for Children," which I'd skimmed previously, because the possibility that my kids could be "in peril" seemed absurdly remote. This time, after chasing my family out to the front porch, I read it more carefully. "Although having a physician for a parent is not a prescription for disaster, there are some perils to recognize."

When I'd finished the article, I put the magazine down on the kitchen table. It was obvious there were two things I needed to do: I had to get good sleep when I was working night shifts. And I needed to get some help. The part about getting sleep would be easy. I could stay in a hotel if it came to that. It seemed extravagant and self-indulgent, but it was better than chasing my family out onto the front porch. The second part, getting therapy, was a harder step for me. It's not like I had never seen a therapist before. After Sarah was born, Sally and I went to couples' therapy, and that had been helpful. Working on a marriage after a baby is born with Down syndrome seemed like good preventive maintenance. But me, personally? Getting therapy?

I hesitated because getting therapy seemed to be an admission of a deep flaw in my personality. I'm embarrassed to admit it, but I also worried that it would seem effeminate—not something a real guy would do. I wished they had a more palatable name for it; something like "Getting a guy to show you how to keep from making the same mistake over and over."

The idea of therapy was unappealing, but I couldn't hide from the fact that I was miserable when I failed to get enough sleep if I was working the night shift. I was also making my family miserable, month after month.

I put the bag of carrots away, and wiped off the table with a sponge. *Maybe I should call Karen, the co-pastor at church.* She'd been helpful after Mr. Kelly died after I'd sent him home. And if this problem looked too big for her to help with, maybe she could refer me to a therapist. I called the church. Karen was there, and said I could come over right away.

I went outside and told Sally where I was going.

"Good." She rubbed her hand against my arm. "Good."

Karen referred me to a guy named David Townsend. His office was a few blocks from our house, in a yellow house with a green roof. Jasmine vines twined up the turned porch columns. In the waiting room, I looked at the notices thumb-tacked to the walls: "100% Cotton Meditation Clothes" were advertised on paper that was printed to look like parchment. A neon blue flyer about a workshop in "Polarity Therapy" informed me that "Energy is the vital force in the body." Another flyer said, "Empower yourself with Reiki, an ancient form of Natural Healing." I didn't see any workshops for workaholic fathers of three. There were notices for Tai Chi, Kripalu Yoga, and Zen classes, but nothing about handling stress at work. The only thing I saw for men was a flyer on impotence. At least *that* wasn't the problem.

A chunky man dressed all in black marched into the waiting room and sat in the center of the couch. Black turtleneck, black baggy cargo pants with pockets, snaps, and zippers up and down the legs. Black combat boots, black goatee. I glanced at my watch. He must be scheduled for one of the other therapists in the office. Unless this was David Townsend, and he was using the time to watch me unobserved. Seemed far-fetched, but so did Polar Therapy, Reiki, and the need for a specific set of meditation clothes. Karen wouldn't send me to a therapist who dressed up like a Ninja G.I. Joe. I glanced over at the guy, but he kept facing forward, with a scowl on his face. *No matter how stressed I got at work or at home, I was better off than this guy.*

Feeling better, I looked at the assortment of Celestial Seasonings tea in a homemade rack on the wall. I thought about making a cup, but was afraid it was for the staff.

A bearded guy with close-cropped hair walked out into the waiting room. "Paul?" he asked, making eye contact with me.

"Uh, yeah."

He smiled and shook my hand. "David Townsend. Nice to meet you." He turned, and walked down a short hallway.

I followed him.

In his office, he motioned to a couch as he settled into a chair facing me.

I sank into the cushions, feeling nervous, guarded. When Sally and I had seen the therapist after Sarah had been born, it wasn't like there was a problem with me: the problem was how

Sally and I would deal with our new daughter's Down syndrome. Going to see David was different. By sitting down on that couch I was admitting that *I* had a problem.

I was verbally skillful enough to keep things superficial at first, avoiding anything that would bring emotions into the discussion. I'd go in once a week, and David and I would spar. He'd try to elbow me into a corner with questions about my feelings. I'd dance around, show him some quick footwork, and slip off to the side, peppering him with staccato words of multiple syllables.

I was dazzling, but David was relentless. Of course, he had an edge on me: it was his game, and he'd been doing it for twenty-five years. Workaholics with compartmentalized emotions were nothing new to him.

David seemed inordinately interested in how I felt. I had to learn a whole new syntax to talk with him. Meeting responsibilities? I could talk about that. Getting the work done? I'd been doing that for years. Meeting a goal? I could discuss that with confidence. But whether or not I was happy? It just hadn't come up before.

I don't know what to say about my therapy. Like the conversations you'd hear when telephones were still on party lines, the sneaky pleasures of listening in would soon give way to boredom. I'm embarrassed that the things I learned sound so much like the bullet points in the self-help magazines: before I could take care of other people, I had to take care of myself—I had to get enough sleep, exercise regularly, and eat reasonably nutritious food.

But the real insight was about joy: the amount of joy I'd be able to feel would be in direct proportion to my willingness to feel sad. That was a tough one. For thirty years, I'd been incessantly striving and keeping myself too busy to feel any of the loss and sadness that we all experience from time to time. I'd learned to keep things in tight little compartments. The emotional distance I'd developed in the ER had become habitual, shielding me from negative feelings until they bubbled out as anger.

I'd become facile at the pretense of forgiveness, but I had to learn to really forgive other people, and myself, for the human errors we all make. And as I learned to open up to feelings of joy and sadness, I began to experiment with feeling gratitude.

I started working with David to ensure that I'd never chase my family out of the house again. As it turned out, I became more productive, and happier.

Getting sleep between night shifts proved to be a lot simpler than the therapy. I checked in at the Hampton Inn, a half mile from the house. The relief of standing in that hushed hotel room was delicious, and physical. The air conditioner quietly hummed, and a fringe of light glowed softly at the bottom of the drapes pulled across the window. I hooked the DO NOT DISTURB sign on the door, closed it, and slid the chain lock in place. Sally was the only person in the world who knew where I was. No one would call and no one would knock on the door. I stripped out of my scrubs, took a shower, and tossed the damp towel onto the countertop rather than hanging it up on the rack. I was, after all, in a hotel. The sheets were crisp and clean and unslept in. I slipped into bed, and went to sleep, like a load of gravel sliding off the back of a dump truck. At one o'clock, I woke up, hungry. I walked across the street to Shoney's for lunch. Back in bed, I stretched, and felt guilty pleasure as I drifted back to sleep. I woke up at five o'clock, shaved and showered, and checked out of the hotel. At home, Sally and the kids were eating toast, yogurt, and carrot sticks for supper. They were doing fine, and seemed glad to see me.

"Want some yogurt?" Sally asked.

"Thanks," I replied, "but I was thinking I may eat at the Broad Street Diner." I was on a roll. A man who sleeps at the Hampton Inn doesn't eat raw carrots and yogurt.

"Sounds good," Sally said, smiling. "Take a book."

I felt a rush of gratitude for Sally's generosity. I still felt guilty, eating out while Sally and the kids were eating at home. But Sally and I had talked about it, and she'd encouraged me to go ahead and indulge myself. "Buddy," she'd said. "Night shifts suck. You should do anything you can to make them better."

She's always known that people should take care of themselves. Sounds selfish saying it, but I've come to think it's true. I was glad that she took dance classes, and joined book clubs, and I encouraged her to take yearly vacations with three close friends she'd made, working in an ICU twenty years earlier. But I used to resent it when Sally got a babysitter just to get some time to herself. I'd be scheduled for a 3–11 shift, knowing I'd get my ass kicked at work, and Sally would mention she had a babysitter because she needed to take a break. But to go out for dinner by herself, while I was clawing my way through a shift?

I imagined her tucked into a booth in the corner of Elmo's Diner, sipping a glass of Pinot Grigio. She'd open her book and smile contentedly. *I'd be in the ER, twelve charts behind.* She'd have a leisurely meal, glancing up from time to time to thank the waiter when he filled her glass with water. *Patients would be mad and EMS squads would be lined up at the loading dock.* She wouldn't have dessert at the diner. She'd stroll down Ninth Street to Francesca's, a little dessert shop, and have a scoop of sorbet. Probably raspberry champagne. *About that time, I'd be doing a rectal exam on a GI bleeder.* She'd keep reading, until she was sure the kids were in bed, asleep. *If I really hustled, I could clear out a twelve-minute space to wolf down my food.* Then she'd go home, pay the babysitter, set up the coffee for the next morning, and get into bed with her book. *I'd be in the ER, wishing I had time to pee.* She'd read till she got sleepy, then doze off. *I'd still have an hour to go before I could leave the ER.*

But after I'd slept all day in a hotel, she was suggesting I go out to eat while she looked after the kids. Gratefully, I went to the restaurant, ordered my food, and read *Get Shorty*. I glanced up, from time to time, to thank the waiter for refilling my coffee. I enjoyed this reprieve from the demands of work and family, and finally understood why Sally had needed time away. When I worked the afternoon, late evening, or night shifts, I wasn't there to help with the bedtime routine or the breakfast routine—I got to bed late and slept late. For a significant part of each month, Sally functioned as a single mom. Or worse, a single mom with a sleep-deprived ogre upstairs, ready to spring out of bed at the slightest noise. As I gained insight, I saw that she'd been struggling for years to mitigate the effect my shift work had on our family.

After supper, I went to a local health food store and bought a pound of dark roast coffee and made a salad at the salad bar. I went to work that night well rested and well fed. I brewed a pot of the gourmet coffee, and left a note by the pot so people wouldn't think the coffee was stale just because it was darker than usual. I enjoyed sharing the small treat of good coffee. When Dr. Holt came down to the ER for an admission, I offered him a cup. "Magnolia Grill Blend," I said. "Fresh pot." He followed me back to the small break room adjacent to the locker rooms.

"Thanks," he said, toasting me with the cup, and took a sip. "Delicious."

Ricky, the respiratory therapist, liked coffee, so I gave him a cup. The ward clerk, nurses, everyone seemed to like the special coffee. It's become a trademark. "Dr. Austin's on duty," someone will say. "We'll be drinking *good* coffee tonight."

As I started getting solid sleep and treating myself to a pleasant dinner and an Elmore Leonard novel at the start of each night shift, I began to hate night shifts less. Sally and the kids noticed the difference. I was happier. They enjoyed being around me.

I don't know why it took me so long to figure out I'd have to treat myself better if I planned to stay at such a stressful job. When I was a carpenter, I kept my tool chest filled with Craftsman tools, the best I could afford. I kept my chisels sharp: I could shave the back of my wrist with them. And I knew that every dollar I invested on tools, I'd get back. I finally came to think that if I had to spend $60 a day on a hotel just to sleep, in order to keep my job, fuck it. Pay the money. I could see it as an investment in job longevity—a cost of doing what I do. Other people who work rotating shifts may not have to go to a hotel to sleep, but I did. And if it would keep me in harness for another ten years, it was a bargain.

I work between two and five night shifts a month. Usually three. Sleeping in a hotel cost $180 a month. That's $2,160 a year. It would buy a set of braces for John, a family vacation, or a couple of writers' conferences for me. I hated spending that much money just to sleep.

Finally, Sally suggested I sleep at her mother's house in Chapel Hill, about twenty minutes away.

"Would she mind if I just came in and went right to bed?" I asked my wife. "I wouldn't feel like making small talk."

"You should ask her."

The next time Sally, the kids, and I went over to visit, Betty asked me if I wanted to sleep at her house when I was working night shifts.

"I'd love to," I said, "but I'm not very good company when I'm working nights."

"Don't worry about that," Betty said, gesturing toward the door. "You could just let yourself in and go right upstairs."

As it turned out, it was even easier than staying at the Hampton Inn. I'd get there between eight thirty and nine in the morning and whistle as I let myself in, so I wouldn't scare her. She'd whistle back, and I'd tiptoe upstairs. That was it. I could sneak out for lunch and back without talking to anyone.

The house was set back in a heavily wooded lot. As I pulled my pickup truck into the circle drive, I felt as if I were entering a refuge. Geese waddled up into the backyard to eat the dried corn Betty scattered for them. Hawks circled lazily overhead. Beavers gnawed trees into pointed little stubs. And a depleted ER doc stumbled upstairs to sleep.

At Betty's house, I slept soundly until I woke up for lunch. I'd leave, go to a diner, and read a novel as I ate by myself. After lunch, I'd go back to her house and sleep all afternoon. On the first day of a string of nights, I'd still be on a "day" sleep rhythm, but I needed to rest up for the night ahead. I'd lounge around in bed all day at my mother-in-law's, reading, dozing off, reading, and dozing off again. At about five in the evening, I'd get up, shower, shave, and go downstairs. Betty and I would chat for a few minutes, then I'd drive twenty minutes to Durham, rested, ready for my shift. The other docs in the ER envied the undisturbed rest I got at my mother-in-law's, and would jokingly ask if they could sleep there, too.

My mother-in-law helped save my job and my marriage. I've never been comfortable about accepting gifts, or favors. I'm always afraid I'll be asked for more than I'm willing to give in return. But Betty never asked for anything and didn't mind my coming and going like a house cat. Once I started getting enough sleep, making exercise a priority, and eating well, I found that I was also glad for Sally to take time for herself. Not just for dance classes or the book clubs, but to have a couple of hours to relax and read a detective novel.

I still don't really understand what I learned during that period. I know it involved opening myself to the feelings I'd always suppressed—mostly sadness and loss—in order to experience the joy. As I gave myself permission to pull away from my family when I needed to, trust, intimacy, and laughter began to flourish.

SLEEPING QUARTERS

"Sally, I'm thinking about building a garage." We were lying in bed together, eating Rocky Road ice cream from small bowls. "It would have a room upstairs for when I'm working night shifts."

"Hmm." She took a bite of ice cream.

"Sleeping at your mother's house is great, but I'm afraid I'll doze off on the way over there."

"Driving when you're sleepy is miserable." Sally looked up from her novel.

"If I build it myself, we could pay as we go. Wouldn't have to borrow any money."

Sally took another bite of ice cream.

"Put it in the back of the side lot."

"You plan to build it yourself?" She knew I'd done a fair amount of carpentry. I'd extensively remodeled the first house we'd bought, and had done work on every house we'd had since.

"Yeah," I said. "It'll be fun. And the kids would learn about house construction—see how to dig footings, pour concrete, frame walls, all that stuff."

"Sure," she said. "Go ahead." Sally paused, and then went

back to her book. Maybe she was counting on this being one of my passing enthusiasms.

The next day, I went to Lowe's and thumbed through a catalogue of plans for garages. I stopped when I came to the picture of "The Studio." Tucked under trees and surrounded by shrubs, it looked more like a cottage than a place to park a car. Two dormers looked out over the curving driveway that swept up to the front of the building. The interior view of the studio on the second floor caught my eye. The angled ceilings gave the room an attic-like feel of secrets and seclusion. At the far end, swag curtains were pulled back to reveal mullioned windows. Bookshelves lined one wall, and a barrister's chair and ottoman rested on a Persian rug. I knew that I was staring at perfection.

I bought the catalogue and took it home. In the kitchen, I made a cup of coffee, and leafed through the other pages to make sure I couldn't find a better garage. But I knew I wouldn't: Just as a puppy chooses its owner, this garage had chosen me. It was large enough to engage my imagination, but small enough for me to build. And the upstairs would make perfect sleeping quarters.

Sally came in with the groceries.

I helped her put them away. "I found a book of plans."

"Plans?" She paused with a quart of milk in her hand.

"For the garage," I said.

"Oh." She placed the milk in the refrigerator door. "See any you like?"

"There's one I like a lot." I was eager to show her my favorite, but wanted to wait till the groceries were put away. Like a kid talking his mom into letting him keep a dog, I had to wait for the right moment.

"Which one is it?" she asked, picking up the book.

"Right here," I said. "The Studio."

"Pretty," she said.

I pointed to the dormers in the front. "Those would be tricky, but I bet I could do them."

"When do you plan to start?" She handed the book back to me, and put a couple of cans of tuna into the pantry.

"I don't know." I stared at the picture. "I'd have to order the plans, get building permits, all that stuff." I was halfway hoping Sally would object: I'd enjoyed talking about it, but I wasn't sure I could do it.

The plans, rolled up in a cardboard tube, came in the mail. I slid them out onto the kitchen table. I'd been a construction laborer after quitting college, and had always envied the guy who got to hold the plans. I was finally that guy. I turned to the second page, which showed the dimensions of the building, the details of wiring and insulation. In the far right corner, close-ups of the footings and foundation were drawn, as well as the detail of the rafters nailed into the top plate of the wall. I placed coffee cups on each corner to keep them from curling up, and stared at the clean black lines that showed walls, elevations, and dimensions. When I was a firefighter, my part-time job was doing carpentry work, mostly trimming out show-room spaces at the furniture market. And I'd half-built a cabin out in the woods. But I'd never framed a real house.

Sally and I went to the side yard, and used a garden hose to mark off the garage, 24 feet by 24 feet.

"Big," Sally said.

I nodded.

She looked at her watch. "Time to pick up the kids." She patted my arm. "It's exciting."

I sat in a webbed lawn chair and stared at the snaky green outline of my garage, savoring the idea of building it myself. It would redeem the cabin in the woods I'd left unfinished, and it would provide refuge from the work I did in the ER. The garage would give my life a grand new endeavor—like Michelangelo's chapel, or Noah's Ark.

Later, Sally pulled into the driveway with the kids.

"Come see," I called out to the children.

They ran over. Sally followed.

"That's where the garage is going to be." I pointed to the outline of the hose.

"What's the hose for?" Sam asked. He was three at the time.

"It's the outline of the garage."

"It's going to be nice," John, the curious five-year-old, said. He stared at the hose.

"I'm going to build it myself," I said.

"Cool." John stuck out his bottom lip and nodded. "Think I'll get a snack."

Sarah followed her brothers.

"*I'm* impressed." Sally laughed, hugging my shoulder. "Want some ice cream?"

The next day, when the kids got home from school and day care, I was grading the site with a Bob Cat, a miniature bulldozer I'd gotten from a rental place. The idea is that you shave off progressive layers of soil, until the ground is smooth and level. Turns out it was trickier than it looked when the guy at the rental place showed me the controls, but I could spin around right and left, and go forward and backward like a champ. After working all day, the ground was approaching level. The Bob Cat was a jarring, noisy thing to drive, but, man, it was fun.

John, Sam, and Sarah stood in the grass and stared at the raw dirt I'd scraped flat with the machine. Sally stood behind them.

I switched off the Bob Cat. "Anyone want a ride?"

John dropped his book bag and stepped forward.

Sally smiled uncertainly.

"Climb in."

John clambered up and sat in my lap.

"We're not going to go very fast," I said, as I turned it on.

"Good," John said.

I drove around the site, showing John how quick it could turn. John laughed, and tightened his grip on the bars of the driver's cage.

The city never paved the short street that runs along the side yard, and it has no traffic. I pulled out into the dirt road.

John turned his head, and looked at me.

"Let's see how fast it'll go," I said.

John nodded.

I sped it up, and the Bob Cat zipped along the dirt road.

John laughed loudly.

At the junction of the dirt and paved roads, I looked for traffic, and then eased out past the stop sign. It would probably go faster on pavement.

"You sure this is okay?" John asked.

"Sure," I said. "Let's ride up to Dale's house, see if he's home." Dale lived about three houses down. We scooted up to his house, but no one was there. I was disappointed, because he likes building things too, and I knew he'd be jealous. We turned around and came back.

Sam and Sarah both took turns. Sally didn't want to. Go figure.

That night, sitting in bed, Sally put down her book. "I never would've guessed I'd marry a man who'd ride his kids around in a Bob Cat."

"It was *fun*."

"I know." She laughed. "I'm glad I married a man who'd ride around in a Bob Cat. Just wouldn't have predicted it." That year, our Christmas picture was of the Austin family, sitting in the bucket of the Bob Cat.

When the gravel was delivered, John and Sam ran up the pile over and over, their feet slipping and sliding as the rocks cascaded down with each step. John helped spread the gravel, his little muscles bunching up as he raked the gravel smooth. When the concrete floor was poured, they used it for tricycle and bicycle races. As the second floor got started, I built a ladder from two-by-fours, with a hinged piece of plywood that would lock down over the rungs, to keep the kids from climbing it when I wasn't there. While I was working, I'd let the kids keep me company, or drive nails into a scrap piece of two-by-four.

The garage became a part-time job and a full-time obsession.

Neighbors walking past would wave and sometimes stop to chat. I worked through the summer, autumn, spring, and on into the following summer. Building permits are only good for one year, so I had to go to City Hall to get an extension. I planned to do all of the work myself: drive every nail, run every wire. But as time ran out on the extension, I had to hire out the plumbing, wiring, Sheetrock, roofing, and vinyl siding. But the carpentry I did myself, and as I did it, I felt fully alive.

Working alone most of the time, I felt like Robinson Crusoe, forging a new future with my own hands. Of course, Robinson didn't have power saws and pneumatic nail guns, but he didn't have to work rotating shifts in an ER, either. I liked working in the summer, my skin tanning, a baseball cap to keep the sweat from dripping onto the inside surface of my glasses. I liked working in the winter, my breath visible, staying warm by working, and having a hot cup of coffee, listening to the radio, sometimes country western, sometimes the classical station.

It was my Taj Mahal, my Eiffel Tower, my epic poem to a good day's sleep. I soundproofed the second floor, and put in a full bath, with a tub and shower enclosure. White tile floor in the bathroom. Cedar trim. I put in oak floors and a wood-burning stove.

During the second winter, I was fitting cedar pieces in over the shower enclosure. I used a propane heater, to keep my fingers from getting numb and clumsy. I heard a hissing noise coming from the connection to the tank. *Damn.* I was wanting to get on with the trimwork, instead of fiddling with the heater. I gave the nut a twist to tighten the connection. But I twisted the wrong direction. A huge ball of fire bellowed out, knocking me back. The yellow flames boiled out of the tank, lapping up against the wall. I grabbed a two-by-four and pushed the tank into the center of the room. I worked methodically, pushing slowly against the bottom of the tank, to keep it from toppling over. The fire roared. I was afraid the tank would heat up enough to make the liquid propane boil, which could make the damn thing blow up. BLEVE stands for boiling liquid evaporation vapor explosion. I'd learned that on the fire department.

I ran downstairs, grabbed the hose at the side of the house, turned on the water, and ran back up to the landing on the second floor. I squatted at the door, hiding behind the doorframe, hoping it would shield me from most of the blast if there was an explosion. As I sprayed water onto the tank to keep it cool, I called out Sally's name.

She ran out into the front yard, clutching her robe closed at her chest.

"Call the Fire Department," I yelled over my shoulder.

"What?"

"Dial 9-1-1," I yelled again, turning back to keep the water on the propane tank.

A few minutes later, I heard the sirens of the fire trucks. I began to relax.

By aiming the water at the connection at the propane tank, I could turn the huge ball of fire into a small blue spit, sputtering in the stream of water. But as soon as I took the water away, it blossomed again, giving off a deep *whomp!* sound. I kept the water aimed at the connection, pulling it away from time to time to see if the fire was out. Each time I pulled the stream to the side, the yellow ball of fire sprung to life. The last time I pulled the stream away, nothing happened. There. It was out.

I walked to the house, to call the fire department to say they didn't have to come after all.

"The fire chief will have to inspect the structure," the dispatcher told me. "But if you're sure it's out, I can turn the trucks back."

"I'm sure," I said. "Thanks." I noticed little wisps of burnt hair floating away from my face. I went to the bathroom to look in the mirror. My face was red, and I looked like a cartoon character who'd smoked a cigar with a load in it. My hair was melted into a frizzy fringe, my eyebrows and mustache singed back to half their size. The hair on my arms was gone.

"Are you okay?" Sally said, covering her mouth to stifle a laugh.

"Yeah." I winked. "I'm fine. But I better go wait for the fire chief." I went to the garage, and looked at the puddle of plastic and aluminum that had melted off of the control panel of the heater and burned into the oak floor. Water stood in shallow puddles across the floor. *Damn*. I went back downstairs.

When the fire chief arrived, I took him upstairs. He stared at the scorched propane tank.

"I put it out with the garden hose."

He nodded, then reached down to touch the propane tank, to check if it was hot. He lifted it up with one hand. "Empty," he said.

"Oh." I hadn't put the fire out—the tank had just run dry.

"Going to be nice up here." The fire chief looked around the room. "Mother-in-law room?"

"No," I said. "I work rotating shifts. Need a place to sleep when I'm on the night shift."

"Ahh," he said, his eyebrows up. "A little pout house."

I grinned. "No point in suffering, just because I'm in the doghouse."

"Get you a little fridge up here, put a wide-screen TV right there," he pointed to the sloping space between the dormers. "You'll have it made." He walked back to his car, talking into his walkie-talkie as he went.

Sally and the kids came up. Sam stayed close to Sally. He looked from the ruined heater to me, then back to the heater.

John walked over, and squatted to look. "Did it burn the wood?"

"I don't know." I took out a chisel from my tool belt, and pried a lump of molten metal from floor. "Yup, looks like it scorched it pretty good." I scraped down through the blackened wood until I got to an unburned part. "I can probably sand most of it out. And if a little still shows, it'll just make a better story."

John looked up at me. "Are you okay?"

"Yeah." I shook my head to make short, burnt wisps of hair fly off into the air. "Pretty funny, huh?"

Sarah laughed loudly. "You look like a cartoon man."

We went back inside.

"I was helping Sarah brush her teeth when I heard you calling," Sally said. "I thought you wanted me to come admire some tricky woodworking thing you'd done, and I wanted to get the kids ready for school. Then your voice got louder, and it sounded like you were scared."

"I was."

"You should've heard me talking to the 9-1-1 lady. She asked if anyone was in the structure, and I said my husband was trying to put out the fire with the hose, and the lady said, 'Tell him to leave the structure immediately.'" Sally laughed, and pretended to hold the phone to her ear, then pull it away to stare at it, then put it back to her ear. "I told the lady, 'Okay,' but I was thinking, 'Yeah, right. *You* tell him that, lady.'"

I chuckled.

"Then I told the kids to go to the windows because the fire trucks were coming."

I started laughing.

"Well, I was afraid one of them would hear the sirens and run outside and get squished by a fire truck. So I told them to go to the windows."

"Did they?"

"Oh, yeah," she said. "They were disappointed when the fire trucks didn't show up."

Once I could sleep in the garage, I started hating night shifts less. But it was still hard to sleep during the day before the first night shift, because I was still on a daylight cycle. I'd usually run an errand or two, exercise, then at about eleven fifteen treat myself to an early lunch so I could get home for a nap in the afternoon. One time I invited Sally. Instead of going to a cheap restaurant, I took her to Parrizade, one of the best restaurants in the area. It reminded me of a New York restaurant. The tables were a little too close together and the place was noisy, but the food was really good.

Our first "pre-night lunch date" was in the spring. We sat outside under a canopy of ornamental pear trees, the blossoms white against the blue sky. The waitress brought a small bowl with a grated Reggio cheese and spices, then made a little ceremony of pouring in olive oil. "For the bread," she said, smiling. Sally and I ate the soft bread with the thick crust, sipped wine, and read paperbacks, until our food came. Then we sat and talked, enjoying sitting outside and having a glass of wine with lunch. I felt time slow and became aware of my sun-warmed shirt on the skin of my shoulders. I imagined Sally's breasts, snuggled tight in a sports bra, under her oxford cloth shirt. We lingered over decaf coffee. I needed to get home, to sleep for the long night ahead, but wanted to wring every bit of pleasure I could from our lunch. "We need to get you home," Sally said, smiling. "Get you in bed." Her eyes held mine.

"Check, please."

Sally walked with me up the stairs to my sleeping quarters in the garage. At the door, I fiddled with the keys. Sally stood behind me. I felt a furtive, vibrating thrill that came with the knowledge that we both had clear intentions of making love.

My hand trembled, anticipating the feeling of one's body surfing at the beach, when the wave takes you and you've surrendered control.

Inside, Sally pulled off her shirt and bra, and shimmied out of her jeans and panties. She nestled into the leather chair she'd gotten me for Father's Day.

She pulled me to her. After twenty years, the surprises were rare: we knew all the shortcuts. But that day, the languid pace we'd enjoyed at lunch continued. Then, with the afternoon sun streaming through the curtains, we made love.

"I should let you get to sleep," Sally whispered, as she untangled her legs from mine.

My arm had gone to sleep under her, and as she stepped out of bed, I straightened it. "That felt good," I whispered.

"Really good." She smiled, and kissed me on the lips. She dressed efficiently, walked over, and kissed me again. "Sleep well."

I got up, placed the foam boards into the windows to block out the light, and turned on a sound machine that creates a constant background sound, like a waterfall. I opened *War and Peace* from a set of leather-bound books I'd ordered through the mail when I was in academics, trying to avoid burnout by giving myself a treat. I'd been reading it as my "night shift novel" for the last few months. After about fifteen or twenty minutes, I could feel my eyelids drooping. I put the book on the nightstand, turned out the light, and fell asleep.

GUNSHOT WOUND TO THE CHEST

"PAUL, we've got a trauma red tag coming in." Joanne, the charge nurse, put down the microphone to the EMS radio. "Gunshot wound to the chest."

"Red tag" is shorthand for a patient who's critically ill. It's as close to dead as you can get and still warrant treatment. As the attending in the ER, I'd be in charge of the patient until the trauma surgeon arrived.

"Vital signs?" I looked up from a chart.

"Don't know." She walked toward the trauma bay. "All they said was 'trauma red tag.' They sounded pretty stressed."

"How long has he been down?"

Joanne stopped. "You know everything I know."

"Okay." I held up my hands.

"I'll call a trauma code and make sure the room's set up."

I walked with her to the trauma bay and checked the equipment I'd be using. I then discharged a patient and got another patient's work-up started. Once the red tag arrived, I'd be too busy to get anything else done, and I wanted to clear out as much as I could before it got there.

The paramedics rolled in with a businesslike clatter. Barry

gave the report: "Gunshot wound to the chest." He handed Lisa an IV bag. "Fired a guy this morning, guy came back with a thirty-eight."

"Damn," Lisa said. "Where's he work?" She'd been an ER nurse long enough to be casually curious about the circumstances.

"Insurance office," Barry answered.

A firefighter pumped on the patient's chest, while a paramedic squeezed the Ambu-bag, forcing air through a clear plastic tube going down into the man's trachea.

"On three," Barry said. "One . . . two . . . three." They hefted the patient onto our stretcher. Barry pulled the green oxygen tubing from the nipple on his portable tank and tossed it to Joanne, who hooked it to the flow meter in the wall. The portable tank hissed loudly until Barry twisted the green knob on his tank, turning it off.

I pulled my trauma shears from the back pocket of my scrubs and cut through the blue oxford cloth shirt and tweed sport jacket. With each compression, blood bubbled lazily from a hole in the left side of the chest. "Bag," I called, and I listened for breath sounds in the right side of the man's chest as the firefighter squeezed the Ambu-bag. "Bag," I repeated as I listened to the left side. "He's diminished on the left."

If air pressure builds up between the lungs and the inside of the rib cage, the lungs can't expand. The increasing pressure also keeps the blood in the rest of the body from returning to the heart. The quick fix is to poke a needle between the ribs to vent the air that's under pressure. A tension pneumothorax can be rapidly fatal, and you make the diagnosis based only on hearing the story and doing the physical examination. There isn't time to get an X-ray, and a film of a tension pneumothorax is proof of inexperience or incompetence. I'd been an ER doc long enough to know this guy had one.

I glanced at Barry. "Did you needle him?"

"No, he sounded equal when we tubed him."

"Probably went under tension en route." I looked at Lisa. "Gimme a catheter."

I swiped the chest with orange antiseptic solution, and poked the needle between the ribs on the right side of the chest. Air hissed audibly. I removed the metal needle, leaving the plastic catheter in place. One problem solved.

"Bag," I said, as I listened to the left side again. "Better." I draped my stethoscope around my neck. "Airway; Breathing; what do we have for Circulation?" I cut his khaki pants and underwear away and placed a gloved finger on the crease next to the pubic hair. "I think I've got a femoral pulse with compressions." I looked up to the burly firefighter doing compressions. "Stop CPR." The faint bounding under my finger ceased. "Nothing. Continue CPR." Each time the firefighter pumped his heart, I thought I felt a pulse. "Lisa, how many lines do we have?" If he'd transected one of the major vessels going to or from the heart, he could've easily pumped his entire blood volume into his chest. He could use as much fluid as we could give him.

"I'm starting a second." Lisa slapped the man's pale, floppy arm.

"How much fluid has he had?" I looked at Barry.

"This is his second liter."

I nodded that I'd heard. I didn't want to open this guy's chest. In ten years as an ER doc, I'd only done it on dogs, practicing. The trauma team would be there in a few minutes, and push me out of the way. But that was the only intervention that had any chance of helping him.

The idea is that with penetrating trauma to the chest, if you find a hole in the heart and plug it, you may be able to temporize until a surgeon can fix it. I've never seen it work, but in textbooks and on TV shows it looks easy. If I was in a tiny ER where there wasn't a trauma team, it would be clear that I should go ahead and try it. Of course, if there was any hope of it working, it had to be done right now—not later. And the guy on my stretcher had no pulse. He was essentially dead. I had nothing to lose except my pride when the surgeons pushed me out of the way. "Get the thoracotomy tray," I said, as I squirted orange antiseptic solution onto his chest.

"You're going to open his chest?" Lisa looked up from her IV, her eyebrows raised.

"I'm hoping Ben gets here and takes over." I tore the wrapping loose from the sterile tray holding the instruments, and put on a pair of sterile gloves.

Ben Smith, the trauma surgeon, walked in. "What you got?"

"Gunshot wound to chest. No pulse. Had a tension pneumo on the left when he got here. I needled it, still no pulse." I pointed to the left side of the chest, wet and shiny from the antiseptic. "The only other thing would be to open his chest."

Ben walked over. "*You're* going to do it?"

"All yours, big guy." I stepped back.

"Did he ever have a pulse?" Ben looked over to Barry.

"We were pretty sure we felt a carotid when we first got there."

"Gimme a scalpel." Ben popped on a pair of sterile gloves, looked over to me, and shrugged with his right shoulder. "We got nothing to lose." He glanced up at the firefighter doing chest compressions. "Stop CPR." In one long swipe he cut through the skin. The yellow fat splayed open. He tossed the scalpel onto the tray, wedged the tip of a pair of heavy scissors between two ribs, and cut first up, then down. "Gimme the rib spreaders."

I handed him a bulky stainless steel bar with two paddles.

Ben wrestled the paddles into the incision, then turned a crank on the rib spreaders. The ribs gaped open further and further with each twist. He glanced at the firefighter who'd been doing CPR. "Don't do any more compressions." Ben didn't want to take any chances of getting his hands squished between the patient's sternum and backbone. He leaned over and snaked his hands into the chest. They made a slurping sound.

"The heart's empty. Flat." He frowned, his hands working inside the chest. "There isn't a hole." He pulled his hands out. "Look at what's coming out of his chest. Looks like Kool-Aid." A thin, watery liquid, barely tinted pink, dribbled out onto the stretcher. "Bullet must've tagged his vena cava. The IV fluid's running out as fast as it runs in." He shook his head. "There's nothing we can do here. He probably bled out into his chest before EMS even got there."

I shrugged. "Thanks for coming down."

"So," Lisa said. "Are we calling it?"

"Yup."

"Time of death," Lisa called out, "9:57."

"Good job, team. We just didn't have enough to work with."

Ben slowly cranked the rib spreaders. The gaping mouth he'd made of the man's chest closed. When he tried to pull the instrument out, it got hung up on the ribs. Ben levered the spreaders up and down as he pulled, like a man tugging a hatchet that's stuck in a stump. When the instrument was free, he gently placed it on the sterile tray, tossed his gloves in the trash, washed his hands, and walked out to write a note in the chart.

A watery pink stain spread on the sheet.

I walked up to the head of the stretcher and looked at the man's face. He had a receding hairline, with salt and pepper hair. Looked like a businessman. The bloody, shredded clothes looked like they'd come from an outdoors catalogue, full of photographs of healthy people wearing natural fibers. His yellow tie had a Windsor knot with a tight little dimple in the center. It was snugged up to the collar of his blue oxford cloth shirt, which gaped open from where I'd cut it up the center. This man looked as if he should've been in a photograph in a catalogue, smiling as he handed a set of house plans to a carpenter, or sitting behind a desk. He didn't belong on a bloody stretcher in my ER, dead.

The hole in his chest was .38 inches in diameter. A red dot that was bigger than a quarter inch, smaller than a half an inch. "Looks like he was a nice guy."

Lisa looked at me and blinked. "Huh?"

"You know." I pointed to his clothes. "Doesn't look like a gangbanger, or a biker or anything."

Lisa nodded.

Several years ago, I took care of a woman who'd been shot in the abdomen while sitting on her front porch. Drive-by. She was scared. We got IVs in her, got her blood started, and the surgeons took her straight to the operating room. It was a satisfying case because the docs and nurses in the ER did our jobs quickly, and the patient seemed to have the same agenda we had—increasing her odds of survival. But a patient who gets shot while shooting someone else often brings the hostility of the conflict with him. If his wounds are life-threatening, the patient usually cooperates. But if it's a gunshot wound to the leg or shoulder, the anger and bravado that got him shot is often still intact.

"Sir, can you tell me what happened?"

"What's it look like?" The skinny eighteen-year-old scowls. "Motherfucker shot me in the leg."

"Okay." I take a deep breath, and let it slowly out. I've got an hour before I get off work. If a miracle happens, and I can get the films, and get a physician's assistant to clean and dress the wound, I can get out on time and not have to dump this on the doc who's coming on duty. "What did they shoot you with?" A wound from a high-velocity rifle causes more tissue damage than does, say, a handgun.

"What you think he shot me with?" The tough guy snorts. "A gun."

"Pistol or rifle?"

"Pistol." He smirks. "Does it look like I was out hunting buffalo?" He grins and cuts his eyes over to the nurse.

The nurse looks at me with a bored expression. "Want an IV?"

"Sure."

"Naw, you-all can forget about the IV bullshit right here and now." He shakes his head. "I got enough holes in me already without you sticking more in me."

The nurse rolls her eyes. To the eighteen-year-old on the stretcher, it's all a new thing. He's seen it on TV, and now it's happening to him in real life. But to the ER nurse, it seems like the billionth time someone comes in shot, or stabbed, and refuses an IV. She looks at me.

When I first started, I would've spent half an hour futilely pleading with the guy to let us do our job. Now I look at the nurse and say, "Document 'patient refuses.'"

The girlfriend will arrive, pull out a cell phone, punch in some numbers, and start informing friends and family. As often as not, she's our ally, and talks the tough guy into getting his tetanus shot.

If he's sober, it's easy: you make sure he understands the risks of refusing treatment, and give him the choice. Then you document that the patient had adequate decision-making capacity, and that he refused. End of discussion. If he's drunk, you're stuck because he isn't competent to refuse treatment. Then it's a round robin of pleading, cajoling the nurses taking care of him, asking the family or friends to help. And sitting on the stretcher, in the center of all this attention and effort, is the sullen, wounded, petulant King for the Day.

I stood at the end of the stretcher and stared at the dead man lying there, his cotton shirt and tweed jacket open and askew. This was an adventure he'd probably not been looking for. I stared at his face. He didn't look scared, or stunned. As he'd knotted his tie that morning, had he thought about the guy he was going to fire that day? Maybe mentioned it to his wife at breakfast, as he ate a bowl of bran flakes?

Lisa and the nurses' assistant rolled the dead man onto his left side to get him in a body bag. The bag, made of a heavy, translucent plastic, has a zipper running down its length. Lisa tied a tag to his toe, pulled the zipper up to the man's waist, and tied another tag to the zipper. She looked back at me. "His wife's here. In the Family Room."

"I'll talk with her in a second. Anyone call the coroner?"

She shook her head. "Don't think so." She spread a white sheet up over the body bag and tucked it up around the body's shoulders, concealing the primitive colors of our failed resuscitation. After the wife had seen the body, all Lisa would have to do was pull off the sheet, zip the bag up over his head, and send the body to the morgue.

I stepped out to the nurses' station and asked the ward clerk to page the coroner. While I waited for him to call back, I could talk with the man's family. Lisa joined me, and we walked toward the Family Room. "Do we know his name?" I asked her.

"Stevens."

The worst part of my job is telling someone that their husband, wife, son, or daughter is dead. A failed resuscitation leaves the whole team feeling empty and defeated. As I step away from the newly dead body, I feel a hard little nubbin of failure. I always tell the team they've done a good job, partly to honor their effort, but also to console myself. But at that point, the failure is circumscribed—it's either a matter of imperfect technique, a limitation of medical technology, or the predictable result of working on an organism that's too damn dead to bring back to life.

But when I go talk to a family, the tragedy becomes real and undeniable. This wasn't an organism that had failed resuscitation, this was a person. A person with family, and friends. And I've found no words that can ease the pain of the people left behind. If I'm careful and lucky, the way I hand them this unwanted load won't add to their burden. That's the best I can hope for.

I was glad Lisa was going with me to talk to the wife. Lisa's been an ER nurse for years. She's usually direct, often blunt, but gentle when she needs to be. Lisa would stay with Mrs. Stevens after I told her that her husband was dead. That way, I could spring free and keep the other patients moving through the department.

I knocked on the door of the Family Room as we entered. It's a small, windowless room, hardly larger than a closet.

A woman in a navy blue skirt and white blouse stood and looked me warily in the eyes. She clutched a crumpled Kleenex in her hands.

"Mrs. Stevens?"

She nodded.

I gestured to the chair she'd been sitting in, sat down in the one beside it, and faced her.

She sat without taking her eyes off mine.

"Your husband's been shot . . ."

She nodded.

"And in spite of everything the rescue squad, nurses, and doctors could do, we couldn't get his heart beating."

She narrowed her eyes, and nodded again.

"I'm sorry, but he died."

She closed her eyes tight. A tear squeezed from each. Her mouth clamped into a tight, pale line.

Lisa and I waited.

Mrs. Stevens gasped and started to cry.

I touched her shoulder, and she leaned against me, crying.

Lisa rubbed her back gently.

I've read articles and textbooks on how to break bad news. And I often remember how Dr. Nicholson, our obstetrician, told Sally and me that our daughter had Down syndrome. He spoke gently and clearly. Used simple words. He took his time, and allowed us to cry. A doctor's demeanor at the bedside reflects who he or she is, but it also reflects techniques that have been learned, and I've tried to pay attention. I try to be like Dr. Nicholson.

I watch for cues from the family. If they're shrinking back, shaking their heads, saying with every gesture and posture, "I don't want to know," I work around to it slowly, to give them time to prepare. If they're fidgety, and look like they want me to get on with it, I do. As gently as possible.

On National Public Radio I heard a piece once about a woman who played the guitar for people as they were dying. She'd sit with the person's family, next to the deathbed, and play quiet, restful pieces, to ease the journey. Must've been hospice patients. She said she played the person's favorite piece, or pieces by their favorite composer. She talked about the peace, and beauty, the transcendence of the experience. I envied her. There are no candles in the ER. No Bach concertos for the guitar. Just unforgiving fluorescent lights and the squawking of the overhead pager. I can't remember a death that was peaceful, beautiful, or transcendent. Death here is usually a noisy, hurried scramble through a harsh, industrial environment. The clock, like a huge hydraulic piston, relentlessly squeezes until I say, "Unless anyone has any ideas, we'll call this one." A nurse looks at the clock, and clearly calls the time.

"Did he suffer?" Mrs. Stevens wiped her cheeks with the palm of her hand.

Lisa gave her a Kleenex.

"No, he didn't." The certainty in my voice was meant as a kindness. But really, who knows how much we suffer as we die?

"Is there anyone in the family we can call for you?" Lisa held out another Kleenex.

"My son." Mrs. Stevens started crying again. "He's in California."

"Is there anyone who lives close by?"

Mrs. Stevens shook her head and covered her face with her hands.

Lisa looked over to me and raised her eyebrows. We couldn't leave Mrs. Stevens by herself, but we needed to get back to work. Lisa gestured toward the door with her head, letting me know I could leave and that she'd stay.

I wished there was something that would ease her pain, but I had nothing to offer but my presence. I waited. "Mrs. Stevens, do you have any other questions?"

She shook her head without looking up. "No."

"I'll be here for several hours. And you can call later. My name is Dr. Austin."

I went out into the hallway, relieved to get away from the pain and loneliness of the Family Room, back to the clatter of phones ringing and monitor alarms chiming. Three empty stretchers were lined up against the wall; a security video camera stared at me from the ceiling.

I went to the bathroom, took a deep breath, and let it out. I splashed my face with cool water and dried it. Other patients and their charts were waiting for me in the rack. I walked back into the ER.

Someone had already moved the body to another room, to open up the trauma bay. A man from housekeeping was slowly mopping the floor. New suction tubing coiled above the clear plastic canister, and the countertops had all been wiped down with antiseptic solution, ready for the next red tag.

I walked to the chart rack, hoping for a patient with a problem I could fix.

WHY DON'T YOU *DO* SOMETHING?

"Looks good," I said, staring at the dry-erase board listing the patients in the emergency room. At 7:10 on a Friday morning, there were only three names on the board. Rick Earnhardt had finished his night shift and had gone home. I was the day shift doc, and had just taken over the ER.

"Don't say it." Joanne, the charge nurse, held up her right hand.

Slow mornings in the ER can elicit a comment, but nobody in their right mind would actually say the word "quiet." It's almost as bad as the word "slow." As soon as someone says either of those two, the EMS radio squawks with bad news, or a crying mother runs in, clutching a blue and floppy infant. So, part of ER culture is to avoid those words. It's not that we're superstitious; we just don't see any point in taking unnecessary chances.

I grinned at the board, winked at Joanne, and wordlessly went to make a pot of coffee. I had the upcoming weekend off, so I was doubly grateful for a slow start to the day. With a fresh cup of coffee, I went back to the booth where we dictate our reports. Two bookshelves run above two telephones, and they're always a mess: medical texts slumped to their sides, and more books stacked on top of them. Three empty bottles of hand lotion were crowded next to a cup of cold coffee. Disposable paper tape measures were jumbled up with ear curettes and a reflex hammer. I sipped my coffee as I put the books right side up, and threw away the thrash. I wiped the Formica desktops with rubbing alcohol, enjoying the extra clean smell.

Someone else must've used the "Q" word, because just as I sat down, a rescue squad called in: "Durham County EMS Forty to Durham Regional." Behind the paramedic's voice, you could hear the sirens wailing, and an air horn blasting. They must have someone who's in really bad shape.

"Medic Forty, this is Durham Regional," Lisa said into the microphone. "Go ahead."

"We have a forty-three-year-old female who complained of a severe headache, and then went unresponsive." The paramedic was trying for the bored monotone of an airline pilot telling you to buckle your seatbelts, but his voice trembled. "We have an IV. She's nasotracheally intubated. We have an ETA of about eight to ten." The siren yelped and warbled in the background, the air horn blared.

We had eight minutes before they arrived, so I had time to eat half a fitness bar, gulp down some more coffee, and go to the bathroom. When I got back, Lisa and another nurse, Robert, were setting up room 10. I opened the airway box, and started checking my equipment.

"They said she had a nasotracheal tube," Robert told me.

"Yeah, I know," I said, as I clicked the blade into the handle. The tiny bulb at the end was a bright point of light. "But it could get pulled out, or they could've meant she has a nasal trumpet." A nasal trumpet is just a four-inch, flexible rubber tube that flares at one end. If you're using a face mask to ventilate the patient, you can increase the air you push in by sliding a nasal trumpet down one nostril. But it doesn't go down into the trachea, and doesn't begin to secure the airway.

Robert nodded.

"Who's going to be the primary nurse?" I asked. It can get chaotic when a dying patient arrives, and I like to know who's doing what before the patient's in the room.

"That would be me." Robert raised his hand, then tore a narrow strip of tape and stuck it to his scrub pants, where it would be handy when he needed to tape down an IV. He'd been an ER nurse for several years, and I was glad he was in the room. "Laura will be helping me." Laura had just finished nursing school, and had been shadowing Robert, orienting to the department. Five years ago, you couldn't get a job in the ER without several years of experience, but with the national nursing shortage, we're glad to get whoever we can.

"Okay." I nodded at Laura, and smiled.

Jessica, one of the other nurses, walked in.

"You gonna record?" I asked her.

She sighed, and held up her pen. After working with me for several years, she thinks I'm hyperactive and too compulsive, and has told me as much. She has a deep southern accent, and writes with loopy, perfect, curlycue letters.

"Can you get the intubation drugs ready?"

"Do you mind getting the drug box?" she asked one of the nurses' assistants.

We stood, listening to the suction catheter's constant tiny insucking of air.

"I thought they said she was intubated," Jessica said. She

shrugged. "But they could've meant they just had a nasal trumpet in."

"Yeah," I said, checking the balloon at the end of an endotracheal tube. "And sure as shit, if we're not ready, she won't have squat for an airway."

"She's unresponsive," one paramedic said loudly, as they pulled their narrow gurney into the room. "Couldn't intubate her, so we just brought her on in," he added as he unbuckled the orange webbing crisscrossing over the patient. "Sorry."

"No problem," I said, moving to the head of our stretcher. "What was her last blood pressure?"

"She said she had a headache, and fell onto the floor," the paramedic said. "They took her to the couch in the other room."

"Where was she?" Jessica, the recording nurse, asked.

"In a group home."

"She a resident?" I asked.

"No," the paramedic said, unhooking his oxygen bottle. "Think she's the cook."

"What was her last pressure?" I asked again. It sounded like she could be a head bleed. They're usually hypertensive, and I wanted to keep the pressure in the 180 range.

"She has a good pulse," he said.

"Robert," I said, "can you get me a pressure?"

He was busy starting another IV. "Laura," he said pleasantly, "could you get us a blood pressure?"

"Sure," she said. She hurried over to put a cuff on the lady's left arm, and push the button to cycle the automatic BP monitor.

"Can you put her on our monitor, too?" Robert asked, as he slid the catheter into the woman's vein. He's been doing it long enough to enjoy using his "smooth and pleasant" voice.

Laura snapped our monitor leads onto the woman's chest. She looked at the monitor. "Her pressure's 230 over 114," she said.

"Thanks," I said to Laura. "Ma'am," I said loudly to the woman. "You're in the emergency room."

No response.

Her breathing was sonorous. A trickle of blood had run down from her right nostril, from the paramedic's attempt to stick a tube through the nose down into the trachea. I pinched the skin over her collarbone, hard. "Ma'am," I repeated. "You're in the emergency room."

Still no response.

"Okay," I said. "Let's get her meds in, and intubate her."

While Robert drew up the paralytics, I walked to the end of the stretcher and pinched her toes, hard. No response. If it *was* an intracranial hemorrhage that had made her this unresponsive, it was probably a big one, which would make a meaningful recovery unlikely. Of course, you never know, and this wasn't the time to ponder the patient's ultimate fate.

Robert looked over to Laura. "You can push the drugs if you want." He nodded to me. "He'll tell you what he wants, and I'll hand you the syringes." Robert was letting Laura do a little. Nothing that she could mess up; but when you're learning how to work emergencies, it helps to start with simple, uncomplicated tasks. The drugs she'd be pushing would paralyze the patient, to keep her from reflexively struggling against the tube I'd be sticking down her throat, between her vocal cords.

Laura pushed the plunger of the syringes in the right order, and the patient's muscle tone went flaccid. With the laryngoscope, I swept her tongue off to the side, and peered down her throat. There was blood from the paramedic's attempt to place a nasotracheal tube, but the anatomy hadn't been distorted. The epiglottis flopped into view. I pulled up, and there were the cords, forming a white inverted V. I felt a rush of enjoyment. All the energy of a roomful of people was focused on those two bright strips of white. "Gimme the tube," I said, and it was in my hand, then between her cords. "Thanks, team," I said, standing up. "Can you hold this?" I asked the respiratory technician.

She answered by gripping the tube between her thumb and forefinger, the heel of her hand pressed firmly against the patient's cheek to keep the tube from slipping further in, or out.

I listened to the lungs on both sides, and heard the symmetrical *whooshes* of good air movement. The pulse oximeter stayed at 98 percent, and the CO_2 detector showed I was in the trachea. *Cool.*

"Thanks, team," I said again. "Good job." I stepped over the oxygen tubing running along the floor, and ducked under the monitor wires running down from the monitor near the ceiling, picking my way through like a hunter sneaking through a barbed-wire fence. I walked to the door of the room. "I need a portable chest X-ray," I said to the ward clerk.

"Already called them."

I went back to the room. "What's her pressure?"

"220 over 112," Robert said.

"Let's hang some nitroprusside," I said. "Shoot for about 180." Nitroprusside is a potent medication that lowers blood pressure swiftly. It's a great drug, because if the pressure drops too far, you can turn it down and the pressure comes right back up. I listened for the sound of the portable X-ray machine, but didn't hear it. I walked out to the ward clerk's desk again. "I really want my chest X-ray."

"I've called them twice; they say they'll be here."

"Can you get me the radiologist?"

When she had him on the phone, she transferred the call to me. "Hey," I said into the phone. "I've got two problems and I need your help. First, I need a CT. I've got a hypertensive lady who went unresponsive after a sudden headache. She's intubated."

"Okay," the radiologist said, knowing, like I did, this was probably a head bleed and the CT was a real emergency.

"Problem number two: Twice, I've asked for a chest X-ray to confirm tube placement on the head bleed. So far all I've heard is 'They'll get to it.' What I *want* to hear is the *vvvttt-vvvttt-vvvttt* sound of a portable X-ray machine coming down the hallway."

"Got it," he said, and hung up.

I like working with people who don't waste a lot of words. I stuck my head out into the hallway. "Can you page the neurosurgery attending for me?"

Robert checked the patient's blood pressure again.

"Okay," I said. "Are we ready for CT? Because I'm going to raise hell if we have to wait for the CT. I don't want them to come over here, and us be the holdup."

Robert grinned, raised his eyebrows, and looked at Laura.

"What?" I asked.

"Nothing." Robert laughed. "I'd just told her how you get."

"What?" I said, my hands out to the sides.

Everyone laughed.

"Nothing," Robert said. "But have you missed a dose of your Lithium?" That's a medication used for manic patients.

"I quit taking it," I joked. "Made everything seem to move too slow." I turned to Jessica, the recording nurse. "How long have we been at this?"

She looked at her resuscitation record, then her watch. "Twelve minutes."

"See?" I said to Robert. "We gotta keep things moving."

Robert nodded, but gave a slight shrug with his left shoulder.

I probably need to chill out a little bit. But it always feels like you're working faster than you are. Twelve minutes wasn't bad, considering we'd had to get the woman off the paramedic's stretcher, over to ours, get the meds in, and call for the chest X-ray twice. But it's too easy to relax after you have the patient intubated; and if you do ease up, the process expands into half an hour, forty-five minutes, and then into hours, before you know it. So I tend to push push push. I try not to be unpleasant about it, but sometimes things need to be done in a hurry.

"Any family here?" I asked Jessica.

"I think there's a sister in the Family Room," she said.

"Robert?" I asked. "You okay?" I don't like leaving a room if a nurse feels like I need to stay.

"Yeah," he said. "We're good." He was starting to pull down her underwear in order to slip a thin rubber tube through her urethra, to drain her bladder.

"If it doesn't slow us down," I pointed to the patient's crotch, "go ahead and put in a Foley. But if CT's ready, do the Foley when we get back."

"Okay," he said.

As I walked toward Family Room, I glanced at the chart to see the patient's name: Mrs. Auborn.

I knocked lightly on the door, and walked in. An African-American woman who looked to be about thirty-five or forty was sitting in a chair next to a teenaged boy.

"I'm Dr. Austin," I said, holding out my hand. "And you are Mrs. Auborn's . . . ?"

"Sister," she answered. "This is her son, Derek." She gestured to the young man sitting beside her.

I shook Derek's hand and sat, leaving an empty chair between us. I didn't want to crowd them, or have to tilt my head back to see them clearly through my bifocals. "Do you know what's happened so far?"

"They said she had a headache, then fell out," the sister replied.

"Yes, ma'am," I said softly, nodding. "It happened at the group home where she works."

The teenager nodded short, quick nods, as if asking me to get to the point.

"We're getting ready to take her over for a CAT scan," I continued, "because I'm concerned she may have had a blood vessel leaking into her brain."

The sister gasped, and held her hand in front of her mouth. The young man stiffened.

I waited.

"Is she going to be all right?" The sister spoke from behind her hand, her eyes closed. A tear ran down her right cheek.

I looked over to Derek. "I hope so," I said. "But right now, it looks serious. We're doing everything we can." Those words weren't a lie: it did look serious, and I did hope she'd be all right. But other, more honest words came to mind. Words like "huge bleed" and "organ donor." It seemed unlikely she'd have any brain function at all, after a head bleed severe enough to make her that unresponsive. Of course, it's surprising how often doctors get surprised. And doctors can be wrong just as often as anyone else, so maybe she'd recover. Maybe she'd even have a meaningful recovery. Who knows?

Derek sat without moving while Mrs. Auborn's sister silently cried.

I waited to see if they had any other questions.

They both kept their eyes on the floor.

"I'd better go back, make sure things are moving forward as fast as they can." I looked over to her son. "My name's Dr. Austin. If you need anything, let me know."

He nodded, and looked back at the floor.

I felt that we hadn't connected, but I didn't know what to do about it. I walked back to the main ER.

"Neurosurgery," the ward clerk announced over the PA system, "answering a page."

I took the call at the nurses' station. "I just want to give you a heads-up. I've got a lady who's probably had a large bleed," I said into the phone. "Forty-three years old, complained of a severe headache, then went to the floor. Hypertensive. She's getting a CT in the next few minutes."

"Okay," he said. "Call me back when you have the scan results."

"Her pressure was in the 220s when she got here. I was going to put her on a nitroprusside drip, shoot for the 180s."

"Sounds good," he said, and hung up.

When I got back to Mrs. Auborn's room, the X-ray tech stood in the doorway with the film in his hand.

"Thanks."

"Sorry it took so long," the tech said.

"No problem." I slid the film onto the fluorescent view box. The film showed the endotracheal tube was in the right place.

"CT's ready for their patient," the ward clerk called out from her desk.

"Let's go," I said, making a shooing motion.

"Wait," Laura said. "The IV bag."

The IV tubing was stretched taut from the patient's arm to the bag hanging from the ceiling. I hung it on the IV pole attached to the stretcher, and they trundled off to CT.

I went to tell Derek and his aunt that Mrs. Auborn was on her way for a CAT scan, and that I'd tell them as soon as I knew the results.

Another chart was in the rack, and I picked it up. A fifteen-year-old, two or three months' pregnant, with vaginal bleeding. Simple, straightforward problem. For me at least, if not for the patient. Once you've ruled out ectopic pregnancy, first-trimester bleeding means a miscarriage, a threatened miscarriage, or some other less emergent problem. Forty percent of pregnancies have bleeding in the first trimester, and of those, about half have a miscarriage and half carry the baby to term. An ectopic pregnancy is the only cause of first-trimester bleeding that can't be safely followed up by the patient's obstetrician. So, although it's an emotionally sensitive problem, at least from a medical point of view, it's pretty simple.

I tapped on the door as I went into the room. A redheaded teenager was lying on the stretcher, and a woman sat in a chair next to her. I shook hands with the girl, and looked over to the woman sitting in the chair. "I'm Dr. Austin, and you are . . . ?"

"Her mother," the woman said. Her hair was thin, dyed flat black. She didn't look scared, or nervous, or even concerned. Maybe she was hoping this was a miscarriage, and her fifteen-year-old daughter would have a chance to start over. Maybe she was hoping for a bouncing baby grandchild, and her calm face was just a mask.

"I understand you've had some bleeding for the last two days?"

"Yes," said the girl on the stretcher. Her chubby, freckled face gave her a girlish look.

"How many pads are you using in a day?" I asked.

"About two or three?" She looked over to her mother, who shrugged. Neither seemed uncomfortable, or concerned.

"When was your last period?" I asked, glad everything was staying clinical, and that there wasn't a lot of maternal recrimination going on.

"About two or three months ago," she said.

I made notes on the front page of the ER record. So far the girl didn't sound like she was that interested in the pregnancy one way or the other. You can't make assumptions, but her attitude was pretty casual. "Can you remember the dates?"

"Nu huh." She shook her head, and shrugged.

"Approximately?" I asked.

"I don't *know*," she said, frowning.

"It's okay," I said, setting the clipboard on the countertop. I don't see how adult women remember the dates of their periods, much less teenagers. I can't remember to take my daily vitamins half the time. I took my stethoscope from around my neck. "Let me listen to your heart and lungs, then I'll come back with a nurse to do the pelvic exam." I'm not sure why we always listen to the heart and lungs, even if the patient's problem is unrelated to the chest. Just part of what we do. Habit. A rite the patient and doc find reassuring. I listened to her chest, then her belly. I gently palpated her abdomen, just above the first few wisps of red pubic hair. "Does that hurt?"

She winced. "A little bit."

"Sorry," I said, as I pulled the sheet up over her belly. "I'll be back in a second, to do the pelvic exam. Have you had one before?"

"Yeah." She nodded.

I went back to the nurses' station to find a nurse to help me with the pelvic.

Robert and Laura had just gotten back with the intubated headache lady. Robert pulled the stretcher into room 10, and stepped on the lever that locked the wheels in place. "Huge bleed," he said, as he lifted the IV bag from the pole on the stretcher, and hung it on the IV hook hanging from the ceiling.

"I'll be in Radiology for a second," I said to the ward clerk, who nodded she'd heard me. I'd do the pelvic exam when I got back.

The radiologist looked up when I walked into the reading room—a soothing, large room, always half dark, cool, and shadowy. "I was just about to call you," he said, turning back to the sheet of film clipped to the fluorescent view box.

"Damn," I said, looking at the images of the brain. The ventricles were filled solid with blood.

"No kidding," he said. "And there's subarachnoid blood everywhere, too." He pointed to the more subtle signs of extensive bleeding. "I don't see any intraparynchemal blood, though." He looked up at me. "So there isn't much way to guess where the bleeding came from. Could be anywhere."

"Thanks." I clapped him on the shoulder and walked quickly back to the ER. "Neurosurgery," I said to the ward clerk.

She picked up the phone to put the page in.

I walked to the room. "What's her pressure?"

"180 over 96," Robert said.

"Cool," I said. "Don't hang the nitroprusside."

"Okay." He looked over at Laura, and winked. He must've told her he wasn't going to hang the nitroprusside because her pressure was coming down on its own.

The neurosurgeon called back, and said he'd be right down. I went to give Derek and his aunt an update, then back to the nurses' station to find someone to help me do the pelvic exam on the fifteen-year-old. After the pelvic, I'd order an ultrasound, a serum pregnancy test, and a blood type. That way she'd be moving toward a disposition while I waited for neurosurgery to come down to see the head bleed.

I found Brittany, the nurse assigned to the girl's room. Brittany had been in the ER for a couple of months. Like Laura, she'd just finished nursing school. But unlike Laura, she had the air of someone accustomed to being the smartest kid in the class. "Fifteen-year-old," I told her. "Pregnant, vaginal bleeding."

She shook her head as we walked to the girl's room.

The girl put her feet in the steel stirrups, and slid her bottom almost to the edge of the stretcher.

I sat on a low stool at the end of the stretcher. "One more scoot," I said.

She moved half an inch closer.

"One more scoot," I said.

The girl sighed, and scooted down further.

"Good job," I said. "Now, if you can let your legs go out to the sides."

The girl covered her eyes with her hands and spread her legs. A narrow stream of blood ran from between her vaginal labia, down between her buttocks.

I asked Brittany to put a towel underneath her.

I positioned the bright lamp over my shoulder, focused on the girl's perineum, and eased the speculum into her vagina. Another thin stream of blood ran down, making a small red dot on the white terrycloth towel on the floor. I opened the speculum, and saw a tiny pair of white feet, the little legs crossed at the ankles. They were beautifully formed, with impossibly perfect toes. They looked like a little charm you'd see on a preteen's bracelet, or the pieces you see in a Monopoly set: the tiny cannon, racecar, and top hat. A thin umbilical cord protruded out with the legs. A tiny person, half in, half out of the cervix.

"Can I have a container?" I softly asked the nurse, as I got the forceps from the sterile packing the speculum had come in.

"What?" Brittany looked at me.

"A container of some sort," I repeated. I grasped the little ankles with the stainless steel forceps, and gently tugged. I didn't want to tear the legs off, and leave the rest of the body in the uterus.

"What?" Brittany asked again.

I took a deep breath. "An emesis basin, anything." I tugged again, a little harder, with the forceps. If the products of conception came out intact, I wanted something to put them in. At less than twenty weeks' gestation, there is zero chance of survival. That's why women who are less than twenty weeks are seen in the ER, rather than going directly to labor and delivery.

"An emesis basin?" she asked.

The baby was stuck. I didn't pull any harder. "Never mind," I said, and stood up. I pulled the sheet over the girl's knees and legs. "You can scoot up," I said. I took off my bloody gloves and dropped them in the waste bucket, then moved to the head of the bed. "It looks like you're having a miscarriage," I softly said, my hand on her shoulder.

She nodded.

"I'm going to call the gynecologist." I looked over to her mother. "Ask them to come down and help."

"Is there any chance the baby will live?" the teenager's mother asked.

"No," I said. "I'm sorry." I waited to see if she or the girl had any reaction, or questions.

They both nodded, without expression.

In the hallway, Brittany frowned. "Why did you want an *emesis* basin?"

"There were two little feet sticking out of the cervix," I said. "I wanted something to put the baby in if it came slithering out."

"Oh." She stopped, and put her hand to her mouth.

I kept walking, feeling badly for having said it so harshly, but I was irritated that she hadn't been more helpful. You sit between the legs of a young pregnant woman with vaginal bleeding and start tugging at something inside her with a pair of forceps, it should be obvious you may be pulling out the products of conception. And even if she didn't understand *why* I wanted a container, she still could have handed me one. I went to the phone, and paged the OB-GYN resident.

A man's voice yelled from Mrs. Auborn's room. "Damn, man, why don't you *do* something? She's bleeding out her nose, man."

The voice was angry and plaintive. "Why are you just standing there?"

I went in. Derek stood four feet from the stretcher, as if too scared to go closer, too scared to move away. His mother's nostril still had a thin rim of blood from the paramedic's attempt at nasotracheally intubating her.

I walked over to him. "Sir," I began.

"Man," he whirled around to face me. "Why ain't you *doing* anything?" His face was contorted with misery. I couldn't tell if it was fear or anger, but there was pleading in his voice.

"Sir," I tried again. "We're doing everything we can. I've already talked with the neurosurgeon, and he's on his way right now."

The woman's right leg twitched.

"Damn, man," he yelled, pointing to the leg, "her leg's shaking. Why don't you *do* something?"

"Give her ten of vec," I said to Robert. Vecuronium is a paralytic. It would stop the twitching for at least a half an hour. I'd not wanted to paralyze her for that long, because the neurosurgeon would want to examine her, and if her whole body had been pharmacologically paralyzed, he wouldn't be able to. He could get an anesthesiologist to reverse the paralytics, but it's a hassle, and time-consuming. Explaining all that to the angry young man seemed impossible, so I went ahead and paralyzed her.

The woman's sister came into the room and put her arm around the young man's shoulders. "Honey," she said in a calm voice. "They're doing everything they can." She looked over at me. "He can't help it," she said. "It's his mother."

"I know," I said.

The young man stormed from the room, crying.

I touched the woman's sister on the arm. "He can't hear it now," I told her. "But later, when he can, tell him we've done everything possible, as quickly as possible," I looked her in the eyes. "Okay?" I knew she understood. I'd talked with them three times, letting them know we were pushing everything as hard as we could.

"I know," she said. "I don't blame you."

"Thanks," I said. "But right now, I'm thinking about him." I gestured toward the hall, where Derek stood. "No matter what happens, he'll need to know his mother got the best care she could, as quickly as she could." I didn't want him to torture himself in the future, wondering if his mother would've lived if he'd been able to make the doctors and nurses to do their jobs faster.

"I'll tell him." She followed the young man down the hall.

"GYN," the ward clerk called out, "returning a page."

I picked up the phone. "Good morning, this is Paul Austin, one of the ER docs. I have a patient who I think would benefit from your consultation."

That's how I habitually begin a discussion with any of the residents or interns. A couple of years ago, one of the other ER docs and I were talking about how much the residents and attendings hate coming down to the ER.

"You can't blame them," Ken had said. "They're in an office full of patients, or upstairs knee-deep in problems, and we're asking them to come down for yet another problem patient from the ER." He shrugged. "You and I both know they have to come down, and they know it, too. From our point of view, we're begging them to come down. From their point of view, we're *making* them come down. Especially the residents. So, when I call them, I try to treat them like a doctor, not a scut dog. Tell them I think my patient would benefit from their consultation."

"Does it work?" I asked. "Does it cut down on the resentment factor?"

"About half the time." Ken smiled. "And at least I know I've given them the chance to act like a doctor."

"How far along is she?" the intern asked over the phone. Her voice was flat: not hostile, but she wasn't going to be one of the ones who came down happily.

"About a month or two," I answered.

"You don't even know her dates?" she said, incredulous, as if she were quizzing a dull pupil. Every specialty has a quirky fact they insist on the ER doc knowing before they're consulted. The orthopedic residents ask if the patient is right-handed or left-handed, before they'll talk about a patient with a wrist injury. The surgical residents want to know when the patient ate their most recent meal, before they hear about a patient with gallstones. They can be legitimate questions, which the resident could ask the patient themselves. But sometimes they seem to use a question like a card up their sleeve, to delay coming down. Other times, the questions just seem intended to make the ER doc feel stupid for consulting them.

"She can't remember," I answered, trying to stay patient. Maybe the resident was having a hectic morning.

"Let me get this straight," she said. "You've paged me without even knowing the dates . . ."

"The salient fact," I interrupted her, "is that a young woman has a tiny pair of feet sticking out of her cervix. I gently pulled on them, they won't come out. If I tear them loose and leave half the fetus in the uterus, you-all will have more problems than if you come down and take over."

"Okay," she said. "I'll come *down there,* and pull it *out*." A simple enough task, her tone implied. If the ER doc was competent enough to do anything, the gynecology resident wouldn't be bothered with it in the first place.

I found Brittany. "Put a line in her, okay?"

Meanwhile, the neurosurgery attending came down, examined Mrs. Auborn, then pulled an order sheet from the shelf, and sat at a table in the middle of the nurses' station. He began writing admission orders.

I sat beside him. "What are you going to do with her?" I asked.

"Put in a bolt," he said. "Her family asked if there was anything I could do." He shrugged sadly. "I can put in a bolt, watch her intracranial pressure."

He would take her to the unit, drill a hole in her skull, and slip a catheter in through the brain, into the ventricle—a cavern inside the brain through which the cerebrospinal fluid circulates. The catheter would be hooked up to a pressure monitor.

"Will she recover?" I asked.

"No," he answered. "Probably not."

I was sorry for Derek, watching his mother slip away while the people who could do something to save her seemed to stand around and watch. I hoped his aunt could help him understand we'd done everything we could. His mother had become an organ donor when she'd first slumped to the floor.

Brian and Laura wheeled Mrs. Auborn to the ICU. Derek and his aunt followed, their heads down.

* * *

The gynecology resident, an attractive young woman with a perky black ponytail, walked up to me. "That patient needs to go upstairs," she said. "*Now*."

I took a deep breath. The little problem I should've been able to take care of without bothering her was now some big goddamn emergency. I found the teenager's nurse. "Can we get her up to labor and delivery?"

Brittany said, "*Yes*. I'll take her up in a *minute*." The GYN resident must've made her mad, too.

"We don't want a huge ordeal down here," I said. "So the quicker we get her upstairs, the better."

"Okay, okay," Brittany said. "I'll get to it."

The resident was sitting at the counter, writing a set of admission orders. Her attending physician was standing next to her.

"You got a minute?" I asked the attending.

I walked around the corner, and the attending followed me.

"Your resident seemed miffed that I didn't just pull harder," I said. "Was this a weak consult?"

"Oh, no," the attending said, her eyes widening. "Not at all. The last thing I'd want is having her bleed to death down here. We're going to take her upstairs, give her some pitocin, and try to get it out."

"Yeah," I said. "And I didn't want to tear the legs off, leave . . ."

"No," she interrupted me. "You don't want to leave a little head up in there for us to fish out."

"Thanks," I said.

I looked at the to-be-seen rack, which had another three charts lined up. The polar symmetry of the two cases struck me, and I hesitated before picking up the next chart. I went to the bathroom, and splashed my face. The lady with the head bleed was going to the ICU, stuck on a respirator, not quite dead, not quite alive. I thought about the teenaged girl with the tiny fetus being squeezed out by the thick fist of her uterus. Of course, this fetus was doomed, just like the woman with the head bleed. The cells may have still been physiologically active, the mitochondria still as busy as the pistons in the engines of the *Titanic*, the heart still pumping furiously, but futily. For both the forty-three-year-old with the brainful of blood and the tiny fetus, death was only on hold.

As an ER doc, my skills are employed in the first hour or so. I have to bring order to a chaotic tangle of medical and social imperatives. By the time a consultant comes to the ER, I usually know what's wrong and have begun fixing the problem. I've kept the team moving forward, and I've talked with the family. Sometimes, I save a life. But much more often, I get things started. Transition someone from a chaos of unstable vital signs and incongruous information to a patient with a defined problem. After I've done my job, another doc admits the patient to the hospital, and continues the care. But both these patients had gotten stuck between life and death, with no alternative possible.

I went back to the rack, picked up the next chart, and got back to work. The rest of the shift wasn't so bad. A sixty-eight-year-old male with chronic obstructive pulmonary disease. A seventy-three-year-old woman with congestive heart failure. A three-year-old with otitis media. Simple things that didn't challenge me clinically or emotionally.

I got home from work at five, and went to the fridge for a beer. There was a note on the kitchen table from Sally:

The kids and I at the pool. Come join us if you'd like, or just take a break. We'll be home by 6:30. No plans for supper.
Love you,
Sally.

When I'm working the 3–11 shift, Sally usually leaves me a note before she goes to bed. The notes start with a line saying she hopes my shift wasn't too bad. Then she tells me about what she and the kids have done that day. At the bottom of the note I write a reply that she'll see in the morning—something like: "Rough shift, glad I'm home. Love you, Paul." Sometimes I draw several valentines, hurried little hearts to soften the concision of my response. In the morning, she'll get up with the kids while I sleep late. I guess she reads my reply, then throws the note away. Otherwise, we'd be awash in our scribbled attempts to stay in contact when our schedules are out of sync. I'd be seeing her in an hour, so there wasn't any point in writing a reply, but I'd feel bad just tossing Sally's note in the trash. In the small and practical things that make a marriage work, Sally's stronger than me.

I left the note on the table and carried my beer into the bathroom. After a quick shower, I went to the walk-through office that Sally and I share. The room measures 6½ by 7 feet, and connects our bedroom with the rest of the house. With an hour to write, I hoped to capture at least a little of the bewilderment I'd felt about the polar symmetry of the first two cases of the day. I was off duty the next morning, so I'd have time to go through what I'd written, and make some sense of it. I took a sip of beer, and began hammering out the words that I hoped would hold an answer.

When Sally and the kids got home from the pool, they were

still wearing bathing suits, their hair wet with the summer smell of chlorine. Sarah had her beach towel around her shoulders like a shawl, and John and Sam shivered in the air-conditioned chill.

After the kids and I had said hello, Sally sent them upstairs to change.

She leaned over me and kissed my head. "Bad day?" Her hair brushed against my shoulders.

"More confusing than bad."

"Want to tell me about it?" She walked into the bedroom.

"Not right now." I saved the document and shut down the computer. "How was the pool?" I turned in the chair to face into our bedroom.

"Good." Sally pulled the straps of her one-piece bathing suit down to her waist, then shimmied the suit down to the floor. She stepped out, picked up the suit, and straightened, facing me. Her tanned arms and legs contrasted with the pale skin of her breasts and torso. The untanned parts seemed to glow in the early evening shadows of the bedroom. "Sam did a backward flip off the low dive, and John did a jackknife off the high dive."

"How 'bout Sarah?"

"She spent most of the time with her headset on, listening to her music." Sally smiled. "I read most of the time."

"Sounds good." Better than my day, anyway. I took a deep breath in, and let it out.

Sally stood with her shoulders straight, the twisted blue bathing suit still dangling from her hand. "You okay?"

"Pretty much." I wanted tell her about the woman with the head bleed and the tiny feet I'd seen in the teenager's vagina, but didn't want to ruin the quiet perfection of her facing me so calmly in the gentle light. I put my arms around her and pulled her toward me. "How 'bout Elmo's Diner for supper?" I felt the damp coolness of her skin through my T-shirt.

"You're nice and warm." She pulled back to face me. "After the kids are in bed, tell me about your day."

It wasn't that simple. When the kids were in bed, we would be, too. And although I wanted to unburden myself to Sally, I also wanted to feel her skin next to mine. If I started talking about my day, I might not be able to stop. Given the choice, I'd rather smell the chlorine and taste the salt on her untanned skin.

The next morning, I sat at my desk next to a window, which opened onto a small back porch. An herb garden perched in pots along the railing. Rosemary, fennel, basil, and thyme grew in shaggy abundance. Sitting at my desk in the quiet morning sun, it seemed fatuous to suggest there had been some mysterious balance between the cases of the day before. Nothing other than random chance had brought them side by side to my emergency room. Those two cases weren't any more tragic than lots of other cases I'd had, and I'd done all there was to do, so why were they on my mind?

Years later, I came across an essay in the *New England Journal of Medicine* that helped me understand what had bothered me so much about that day. Katherine Treadway, M.D., wrote about her experience as a third-year medical student on a pediatric rotation. She and the intern to whom she'd been assigned were walking down a hallway, when the intern stopped to check on a young patient he'd cared for during previous admissions for cancer. The seven-year-old girl was dying. When the intern walked into the room, the girl's mother stood up. The intern put his arms around her. After a few minutes, the mother pulled away and said, "You know, I never thought I would want her to die, but I want her to die. Somehow, when they said there was nothing more they could do, I pictured her in a field of flowers and she'd just be gone. I never thought it would be like this."

Dr. Treadway, now an assistant professor of medicine at Harvard, tells her students that her intern "taught me a profoundly important lesson that night. Many doctors would have walked by that door because everything had been done." But her intern had taught her that "there was one more thing to do—to go into that room and offer whatever comfort his care and concern could bring, to bear witness to the pain of that family. In the end, it was as important as anything else that had been done for that child. In the long years ahead, if you asked the mother what she remembered of that time, I suspect that one memory would be of my intern holding her."

Maybe that's why those two cases continued to bother me. Derek, Mrs. Auborn's son, wouldn't remember a compassionate ER doctor who had offered a hug and emotional support: he'd remember his mother's nose bleeding and her leg twitching while it appeared as if I'd been standing around, doing nothing. And the girl having a miscarriage may remember that I spent more time with a pair of forceps than I did helping her and her mother come to grips with what they were going through.

Dr. Treadway ends her article with some thoughts about the practice of medicine: "it is an intensely intellectual endeavor, demanding that you learn and understand an enormous body of information and that you constantly update that information as new knowledge becomes available, but it is also an endeavor of your heart. At the same time that you are learning about disease and diagnosis and treatment, you are learning about illness, the patient, and yourself."

I sat at my desk, looking out the back window and thinking about the woman with her brain awash in blood, and the teen-aged girl with the tiny little feet protruding from her vagina. I didn't feel the need to beat my breast and say *mea culpa*: I'd given the best care possible under unforgiving time restraints, and I'd been as gentle as I could.

But next time, could I devote a few minutes just to be present to their pain? I know I'll try.

SOMETHING FOR THE PAIN

A HIGH-PITCHED shriek scaled up and down, piercing the normal noises of the ER: the squawking of the paramedics' radio and the retching of the homeless man in the hallway. I grimaced and glanced over to room 27. "What's in there?"

"Broken leg." Joanne, the charge nurse, said. "Down syndrome." She held out a clipboard.

I liked working with Joanne, who is a small-framed woman with gray-blue eyes and feather-cut hair. Over the years we'd worked together, I'd enjoyed our quick snippets of conversation about favorite books, vacations, and kids. She knew that my sixteen-year-old daughter, Sarah, had Down syndrome, but her tone carried nothing personal. Busy shift.

I stiffened from the unexpected tweak of pain as I imagined Sarah screaming like that. I hesitated to reach for the chart. The paramedics had been hammering us all evening and I was maxed out. I didn't have the reserve to deal with anything extra. But the other doc was getting ready to go home, and I didn't want to listen to the screeching until the next doctor came on duty. Taking the clipboard without comment, I walked to the room. I'd focus on the injuries, get her in, get her out.

"Mama mama mama," the woman on the narrow EMS stretcher screamed over and over. Her left leg angled out to the side, just above the ankle, like a freakish extra joint. Her slanted eyes were open wide, and her crowded yellow teeth overlapped unevenly. I felt for a pulse at the top of the foot to see if the fracture had disrupted the arterial flow; without a good blood supply, the limb wouldn't survive. The pulse rose and fell under my finger, fast and strong. I clicked my pen and marked the spot with a small blue "X."

"Let's move her over." Barry, the head paramedic, grabbed a fistful of sheet under the screaming woman.

"Stop." I looked from him to the heavyset woman standing off to the side, clutching a pocketbook. "You are her . . ." I had to speak loudly to be heard over the incessant shrieking. I tried not to scowl from the noise.

"Sister," she said, in an equally loud voice.

"Paul Austin," I said, "one of the ER doctors." Our conversation was like the ones I'd had as a firefighter in my twenties, straining to talk clearly and loudly enough to be heard over the noisy confusion of a working fire. "I want to give her some pain medicine. Is she allergic to any medications that you know of?"

"Peanuts." The sister shook her head. "Only peanuts." She winced and bent forward slightly with her shoulders hunched, as if the screams were hailstones beating down on her.

"She get hurt anywhere else?"

"No."

"What's her name?"

"Madison."

I walked to the head of the paramedics' stretcher, and gently placed my hand on Madison's chubby shoulder. "Madison?" I patted her arm.

"Mama mama mama." The shrieking didn't change in volume, pitch, or rhythm.

"Madison." I took a roll of fat between my thumb and finger and pinched, gently first, then harder, hoping to get her to focus on what I wanted to tell her. She continued screaming. Her eyes looked like those of an animal with its leg in a trap, understanding nothing of the pain that wouldn't go away.

"Let's give her some Dilaudid and Phenergan before we move her," I said to Lisa, the nurse. I wanted the shrieking to stop, and the pain medication would help.

"You don't want to get her on our stretcher first?" She pointed to the woman's forearm. "She doesn't even have an IV."

"Leave—her—where—she—is." I pronounced each word distinctly. "Start an IV. Give her 1 milligram of Dilaudid and 12.5 of Phenergan. Repeat the Dilaudid if you need to. *Then* you can move her."

The paramedics and nurses stared at me. We usually move the patient from the EMS stretcher to ours before we start working on them. Partly because the paramedics need to clear the scene and get back into service, and partly from habit. But my first priority was getting the room quieter, which required that we get the woman's pain under control. I looked Lisa in the eyes. "IV, pain meds, *then* move."

"Okay." She let out a deep breath, shrugged, and snapped an IV tourniquet around Madison's stubby, fat arm.

I stepped over to the sister. "We'll have her feeling better in just a minute or two. I'll go get her X-rays ordered."

I hurried out of the room, eager to get away from the wailing. I felt bad that Madison was hurting so much, especially since she didn't understand what was going on. But her screaming penetrated in an almost physical way. I was ashamed for feeling more irritation at the noise than concern for her pain, but beneath my crust of irritation was something too complicated to get into at the time. I wrote orders for leg films and put them in the ward clerk's rack.

"What's wrong with her?" Carol, the ward clerk on duty that night, was about my age. She enjoyed a bawdy joke and was pleasantly efficient, so I liked working with her. But she also had a sweetness of spirit that helped to counterbalance the casual cynicism that comes so easily when working in an ER.

"Broken leg." I walked away. If I'd told her that Madison had Down syndrome, she'd have said, "Poor thing," or, "Bless her heart," and her unfussy tenderness would've opened up the feelings that I didn't want to deal with. I needed to get through my shift without seeing any similarity between my daughter and the injured woman whose bleating and screeching made her seem less human.

I walked to the X-ray room. The X-ray technicians are often "travelers," techs who've found they can make more money doing fill-in work through agencies. Some are good, some are bad. That evening, the tech was a guy whose name I didn't know, but he was good. Crew cut, stocky, quick. "Need a tib-fib in room twenty-seven," I said.

"Portable?"

"Sure."

He grabbed a film cassette and slid it into a compartment of the wheeled machine.

"Don't move her till she's had some pain meds."

"Okay." His battered white machine made a whirring sound as he headed for the room.

I listened for Madison's screaming. Quiet. I went into the room.

"I gave her the second milligram of Dilaudid," Lisa said. "Zonked her."

I nodded. "Good."

"Can we move her now?" Barry asked.

"Sure." I moved to the other side of the stretcher and grabbed an edge of the sheet to help pull. "And thanks for giving us a minute."

"No problem."

When we hefted her over to our stretcher, Madison moaned, but didn't open her eyes. Closed, they looked almost exactly like Sarah's baby pictures, slanted inward, almost masklike in their exotic curve. She had a small pug nose like Sarah, and a large forehead. But I doubted that her face had ever been as animated as my daughter's, or could show as much intelligence, humor, and grace. I couldn't imagine Madison knowing every movie Julie Andrews had ever made, or the names of the actors who played the twins in both versions of *The Parent Trap*. I couldn't imagine Madison raising her right eyebrow like Sarah did, when emphasizing an ironic point in conversation. Sarah was in the "high-functioning" class at school, read books for preteens, and could make her own connections between books she's read and movies she's seen. Madison looked liked she'd belong in the "severe and profound" class, maybe "trainable mentally handicapped" at best. These are gradations that no parent would want to learn, but once you have a child with Down syndrome, you'll gladly take what you can get.

I turned to Madison's sister. "How did she break her leg?"

"Fell down the steps of the back deck. The wood was wet and slippery."

After the tech had made the X-rays, I asked the sister the standard questions. Madison was twenty-nine years old and, other than Down syndrome, was healthy. Hadn't hit her head, no loss of consciousness. No other injury. She lived with her parents. I did a quick physical exam, and then turned to the sister. "Let me know if she starts hurting again." With the room quiet, I felt I could relax a little. "It's obviously broken." I pointed to Madison's lower leg. "After I see the films, I'll call orthopedics."

The orthopedic resident returned his page and I described, as best I could, the fractures through the two bones that run parallel, forming the lower leg. I was hoping to relay the information quickly, and move on with my other patients.

"How angulated are they?" he asked.

"About fifteen degrees." Some ER docs are really good at describing X-rays over the phone, using all the correct terms, precisely and quickly. I'm not great at describing radiographic findings, but I've been doing it fifteen years, and I know when a fracture is something I can splint and send out, and when it's so complicated that an orthopedist needs to come down to the ER. The resident physicians will sometimes ask multiple questions, looking for reasons I should splint the fracture and send the patient home without their involvement. Even on a good day, it can be irritating. And in this case, I knew that the resident would have to come down and see the patient, no matter how well I described the fracture. When he came in, he could look at the film for himself.

"Both the tibia and the fibula?"

"One's probably less angulated than the other, but they're both comminuted." "Comminuted" means that instead of a simple fracture with clean ends, there are chips and chunks of bone at the fracture site.

"So, which one is worse?"

"The tibia. I don't have the film in front of me," I said. I was feeling defensive, and his insistence at asking more unnecessary questions was irritating me. "Probably be best if you just come in and look at the films."

"So, you don't know which bone is more comminuted?"

"Look, this ain't a fucking quiz show. If you don't want to come see the patient, you need to tell me now so I can ask your attending to come in." I waited a second, and then hung up. What a day—screaming patients with Down syndrome, ortho residents with attitudes. I looked at my watch. Four more hours to go.

I went back to Madison's room, still frustrated with the ortho resident. "She feeling better?"

Her sister had been sitting in a blue plastic chair. She stood, and walked over to the stretcher. "Seems to be."

"When the orthopedist sets the bones, I'll give her more pain medicine."

The sister brushed Madison's hair from her forehead. "Thanks."

"She lives at home?"

"With my parents." Madison's sister shook her head. "But they're getting old."

We stared at Madison's face.

"I have a sixteen-year-old with Down syndrome," I said. "Named Sarah. We'll be looking into group homes when she gets older."

Madison's sister turned her face to look at me, dark circles under her eyes. "I've talked with Mom and Dad about it, but they're . . ." She shrugged.

"It's hard," I said, looking back at Madison's placid face. "But Sarah's looking forward to getting out of the house, having some independence."

"I think Madison would, too," the sister said. "But my parents are used to her being at home." She looked at my face. "But as they get older . . ." She stopped.

"It's a hard transition." Was she afraid Madison would eventually have to move in with her? I didn't want to sound like a salesman for time shares in a group home, but if I could assuage some of the guilt Madison's sister might feel for thinking about finding a place for Madison, it might help. "When Sarah's brothers graduate from high school and move on to college, she'll finish school and move on to a group home. If she didn't, she'd feel like she'd been left behind."

"I think it would be good for Madison, too," her sister said. "If only Mom and Dad could accept it."

We stood quietly for a moment, and then I went to check on my other patients.

The ortho resident, a tall guy in green scrubs and a short white coat, looked at the films, and went to talk with Madison's sister.

Earnhardt and I sat in our little dictating booth, working on charts. "I had to tighten up on the ortho resident," I said.

"Yeah?" Earnhardt looked up at the resident, then back to the prescription he was writing. "What'd he do?"

"Kept pimping me about an X-ray. I couldn't tell if he was jerking my chain, or if he was just trying to understand the fracture."

He shrugged. "Always seemed pretty reasonable when I've talked to him." He tore the script from the pad.

"Now I feel like an asshole."

"Don't." Earnhardt snapped the script under the clip on the clipboard. "If he didn't deserve it this time, he will the next."

When I walked into Madison's room, the ortho resident was talking to her sister. He ignored me. "We'll pull the bones in line and put a plaster splint on tonight. It'll take a couple of days for the swelling to go down, and then we'll put a cast on it."

"Conscious sedation?" I asked. The orthopedic residents are rarely comfortable sedating a patient for a procedure, and I was offering to help.

"Sure," he said, without looking at me. "That'd be great."

Fair enough. We didn't need to be best friends to get Madison's leg taken care of. I ordered the medication to sedate Madison, while the ortho resident got his plaster ready. We didn't exchange ten words.

When we were done, I went to dictate the chart, still feeling bad for barking at the resident. I knew I'd feel lame trying to explain that the screaming woman who looked so much like my daughter had made me feel vulnerable and clumsy. And I didn't plan to confess my sensation of inadequacy at describing X-ray findings. No reason to get into all that; but I did want to apologize for being an asshole over the phone. But by the time I'd finished my dictation, he'd gone.

* * *

I checked up on Madison a couple of times. Even after the sedation had worn off, her face remained slack and expressionless; her Down syndrome was much more severe than Sarah's. I found this perversely reassuring: My fears that my daughter would someday wail incomprehensibly in an ER diminished somewhat. Sarah would never feel or sound like an animal with its leg caught in a trap; even in pain, she'd still be Sarah, her humanity intact.

Back in Madison's room, I spoke one last time with her sister. "Do you know about the ARC?"

She shook her head.

"The Association of Retarded Citizens." I pulled a paper towel from the stainless steel dispenser over the sink in the corner. "They offer respite care. Someone can come out to look after Madison while you go take a break. They can also help you look into group homes, activities, movies, dances, stuff like that." I clicked my pen. "What about the Comprehensive Chromosome Clinic? Heard of them?"

"Huh-uh."

"It's a clinic with a doc who knows a lot about Down syndrome, a cardiologist, a physical therapist, an occupational therapist, every specialty you need to see, all in one morning." I wrote Sally's and my name on the paper towel. "My wife, Sally, used to work there." I wrote our phone number and address under our names, in clear block print. "Here."

Madison's sister took the paper towel and looked at it.

"Sally keeps up with this stuff better than I do. Give us a call, and if she answers, tell her I took care of your sister here in the ER. Don't worry—people call her about Down syndrome stuff all the time."

I rarely give out my home phone number to people at work, and most of the ER docs have unlisted numbers. We serve a troubled, sometimes dangerous population, and we instinctively keep work and home separate. There's too much turmoil and pain at work to risk letting it spill into our homes. The simple cases aren't so bad—a kid with a laceration on the forehead from standing too close to a swing set, or a guy with a fishing lure dangling from his ear—these are innocent injuries that heal and are over as soon as we take the stitches out. But we see too many examples of long-standing meanness and indifference—guys with their eyes beat shut, women whose boyfriends have given them gonorrhea, kids with diaper rash that's been ignored until the whole perineum is puffy, red, and weeping. It's not surprising that we try to peel away our work, like a pair of gloves, before going home.

A couple of weeks later, I was at home sitting on the back porch, reading *Empire Falls* by Richard Russo, the bill of my ball cap shading my eyes from the last rays of the early evening sun. Sarah had finished her homework and was swinging on the front porch swing. John and Sam were up the street playing with friends.

Sally backed through the kitchen door and onto the deck, a beer in each hand. She was wearing a denim wraparound skirt over a black leotard. She's still taking two dance classes a week. Every year they give a recital, and Sally wonders if she's getting too old to perform, but there are always a couple of the younger ones glancing over at her, trying to keep up. I'm proud she's still dancing. Plus that, she looks good in a Danskin top.

"Beer?" She carried two Coronas, each with a small wedge of lime floated inside the clear glass bottle.

"Thanks." I held my place in the paperback with my finger.

She handed me one of the beers, and with her free hand corralled a big handful of her hair, lifting it away from her neck. Sally's fifty-two, and quit dying her hair about five years ago. She's one of those lucky women with thick, riotous curls of hair that keep looking better as more gray and white streak through it. She calls it "the new blond."

Sally took a sip of her beer. "Did you recently take care of a woman with Down syndrome? Broken leg?" She let the hair flop down over her shoulders.

"Oh, yeah," I said. "Wouldn't stop screaming till we snowed her. I gave her sister our number. Didn't think you'd mind."

"Not at all." Sally sat down in the black metal chair next to mine. "Had a good chat. Gave her a bunch of names and numbers."

"Thanks." I sipped my beer, enjoying the fresh tart hint of lime.

"She said you were really nice."

"I didn't feel like it. This girl was so profoundly retarded." I took another sip of the beer. "Kept screaming and screaming." I shook my head. "I kept thinking how glad I was that Sarah isn't that bad off."

"Sister said you took good care of her."

"Huh." I stared at the wedge of lime. "I gave her the pain medicine mainly to get the room quiet—I was treating myself more than I was treating her."

"Maybe neither of you deserved to suffer."

I looked at her. Even after twenty years of marriage, and even factoring in her background as a psychiatric nurse, I'm still surprised at how much wiser Sally is than I am.

Sarah came out onto the back porch. "When's supper?"

"Soon," Sally said.

"How was work?" Sarah stood by the door. A couple of years ago she would've run right over for a hug, but she'd begun to show a little more reserve during her teen years. I was glad to see that develop. People often tell me, when they discover that I have a daughter with Down syndrome, that "Down syndrome kids are so loving." Their tone suggests that I should be pleased to hear this bit of folk wisdom. But the assertion seems facile. The kind of thing a dog owner might say: "I just love my beagle—he's so calm," or, "We had to get rid of our Scottish terrier; she was smart as a whip, but so hyper." It somehow turns the ability to express love into another stigma of a medical condition, like slanted eyes, decreased muscle tone, or an underdeveloped occiput.

Who knows? Maybe the conventional wisdom is right. Maybe people with Down syndrome do have an easier time showing affection, just as people with autism seem to have a harder time. But I didn't want to view Sarah's affectionate personality as the result of a chromosomal abnormality.

"Work was okay." I held out my arm for an embrace.

She put one hand on her hip and tilted her head. "No hug for you today." She turned, and sauntered back into the kitchen, laughing at the joke she had played on me.

I laughed along, glad that Sarah was confident of our love, and could tease me about it. Underneath my laughter, though, I was vaguely fearful—someday she may lie in someone else's ER with a broken leg, and I won't be there to help. Like Madison, Sarah might have to scream to get relief. But if she has to, I hope she yells and shrieks until someone brings her something for the pain.

THE DEVIL IS A BEAUTIFUL MAN

THE charts of patients waiting for a physician were stuffed, two and three to a slot, in the rack under the clock in the nurses' station. Walking into work at three o'clock that afternoon, I'd threaded my way through hallways clogged with people leaning against the ends of stretchers, slumped over in wheelchairs, and sitting cross-legged on the floor.

"How many are waiting to come back?" I asked Joanne, who was in baggy blue scrubs and white running shoes with navy blue stripes.

"Fifteen, maybe sixteen."

"Anybody need to be seen right now?" I didn't want to start on the routine patients if someone with a more acute problem had just been brought in.

"Not really." She gestured to the rack. "The sickest should be at the front."

I nodded. Starting a shift so far behind can be disheartening because most of the patients are resentful and angry by the time I meet them. You can't blame them—they've been ignored for hours in a chaotic, noisy ER. Their stretcher may be eight feet away from someone vomiting at full volume, with only a curtain between them to filter the deep, gushing sounds of misery. Or they may be next to someone with gastrointestinal bleeding, the rich fecal stench of rotting blood billowing into their space, making their eyes water and stomachs lurch. The ER is a miserable place to watch a clock.

Until I got off duty at eleven that night I'd start each interaction with an apology for the wait, hoping the hard scowls of impatience would soften, the arms crossed tightly over the chest begin to relax—at least enough for us to start talking, the first step in addressing the concern that had brought them in. Then I'd try to move forward through the problem. Even that can be tricky: after waiting for hours, people feel entitled to as much time from the doctor as possible. Every illness has a story, and some people insist that every detail be heard; any attempt on my part to walk in, get the essential information, and then hustle on to the next patient is just further evidence that no one really cares about them.

On a good night, I can take pleasure in shifting gears frequently and smoothly as I move from room to room, patient to patient. On a bad night, I just dig in and hope to dig out, knowing that no matter how bad it gets, my shift will be over in eight hours.

I grabbed the first clipboard and glanced over the paperwork. The patient was eighty-two, and had been sent in from the nursing home for evaluation of a fever. Great. Just great. I'd been hoping for something simple—something I could knock out and keep moving, start chipping away on our backlog. Most nursing home patients have multiple medical problems, and their list of medications can go on for two or three pages. Just sorting out the drug interactions could take hours. Fortunately, that was the nursing home doctor's job, and all I had to do was figure out why my patient had a fever. Still, I was tempted to put the old man's clipboard back, find something quicker. But I'd eventually have to see the patient, so I clicked my pen, noted the time on the chart, and walked toward his room.

Since 89 percent of elderly patients who come to an ER with a fever have some sort of infection, that was the obvious place to start looking. I could almost order the appropriate labs and X-rays without even seeing the patient. The most common infections are in the urinary tract, or the respiratory system, or involve the skin. If I could keep it on autopilot, I could see the patient, quickly get the work-up started, and move on.

Nursing home patients often carry unmistakable stigmata of chronic illness—pale, skinny legs are drawn up into an inflexible fetal pose, and a clear plastic tube snakes out from under the adult diaper, draining an opaque sludge of urine. As often as not, synthetic lamb'swool booties have been strapped to their feet to protect them against the bedsores that form under the unyielding pressure of immobility. The bare toes extending past the booties have thick yellow nails that need to be trimmed.

So, I was surprised when I met my patient: an alert man, with carefully parted white hair. He wore a dark blue robe with baby blue piping that matched his eyes. Sitting propped up on the stretcher, he looked more like a well-rested guest on an ocean liner than a man marooned alone in an ER. His large, knobby hands were folded in his lap; his legs were crossed at the ankles. He wore cordovan leather slippers.

"I'm Paul Austin, one of the ER doctors. I'm sorry you had to wait." The old man's handshake was firm, and brisk.

"You-all are busy." He smiled.

"Durham on a Friday night." I smiled back, grateful for his understanding. "How can I help?"

"Don't know, Doc." He shrugged his shoulders. "I feel fine. The nurses out at the rest home said I have a temperature."

I pulled the stool closer to the stretcher, sat down, and asked him questions about coughs, nausea, vomiting, diarrhea, and urination with burning. He answered each in turn. As I finished the physical examination, I told him we would check some labs and a chest X-ray, and then come back and talk with him.

He nodded. Then softly, pleasantly, he said, "My wife died."

I stopped.

"She was sick for four years. Last year, she was in the hospital over 300 days—302 out of 365. She kept saying she didn't want to go to a nursing home." He looked at the wedding band on his finger, and rubbed it with his right thumb, as if to polish it. "I took those vows, for better or worse, in sickness and health, and I've kept them. I've walked that fiery path." He looked back at me. "I had no idea it could get so rough. I never did put her in a nursing home. I stuck by those vows, but it was hard. Each and every day was hard."

I wanted to take a minute to listen, to offer more than the thin sliver of time his problem required. But I can rarely sit for more than a minute or two, unless I'm telling someone bad news. If someone's just died in the ER, and I'm talking with their wife, or children, or father, I'm obligated and forgiven for squandering a few minutes on a problem that can't be fixed. Otherwise, I need to keep moving. When the ER's clogged, I have an abiding fear that in the waiting room there is a young woman with "routine vaginal bleeding," who actually has a pregnancy in her fallopian tube, and it's about to rupture, causing her to bleed to death. Or maybe a man with a "routine headache" has meningitis, an often fatal infection of the brain. Meanwhile, I'm chatting with a patient.

"Nine days ago, she passed on to glory," he continued. "It was a beautiful funeral. My daughter set it up, and it was just like my wife would'a wanted it. And then three days later, I was in this very bed in this very emergency room, having a mini-stroke. That's when I saw a vision of the devil on that wall right there." He pointed toward the opposite wall, his bony wrist sticking out past his pajama sleeve. "It was plain as day. And he's a beautiful man. He's an archangel. The Bible tells you he's a beautiful man, and it's right. He just glows." The old man put his hand back in his lap. "And just when I was seeing that vision, a preacher friend of mine came to visit. He said, 'Hold strong, 'cause you're walking that fiery path.' That's exactly what he said, 'You're walking that fiery path.' And I said, 'I know I am, and the devil is on the wall right there.'" The old man paused. "This preacher stands six foot six inches tall. He's been married fifty-seven years. Him and his wife's first home was an old chicken coop in Winston-Salem. But they stayed with it, and they're married to this very day."

I liked the old man. The rackful of charts could wait for another minute or two. Joanne was good, and she'd call for me if she needed me.

The old man stared at the white tile wall as if he expected another vision. Then, softly, he began to talk again. "Well, when that preacher walked into the room, the devil just faded off that wall like he hadn't never been there. And I ain't seen him since."

The man's eyes looked straight into mine. "But I've kept walking that fiery path. I'm walking it, and I kept those vows, but I never knew anything could be so hard." He looked away, to the wall, then down to his hands in his lap.

"Sounds like you did the right thing," I said, staring at the blank wall. I admired the way he'd stood up for his wife, but I didn't know what to think about his vision of the devil. The old man spoke with such calm and clarity, I hesitated to ascribe his vision to dementia. Maybe it was from the high fevers he'd been having, or the stress of his wife's death. Meningitis was possible, but there were no other signs to suggest it, so I couldn't see doing a spinal tap. Other than the vision of the devil, his mental status had been absolutely clear. And who's to say? Visions of Jesus have been seen in pancakes and tortillas; why not the devil on a tile wall? "I've got to get your work-up started," I said, "but I'll be back to talk with you soon."

I scribbled the standard orders for the evaluation of a fever of unknown origin. His hospital chart came up from medical records. He'd been spiking fevers for the last six days of his hospitalization. He'd been running a fever when they transferred him to the nursing home thirty-six hours earlier. His blood cultures and urine cultures were all negative.

When his labs, urinalysis, and chest X-ray came back normal, I went back to talk with him. "Sir, I'm not sure why you keep having a fever. You don't have pneumonia, or any other serious infection I can find. I think it's okay for you to go back, and I've spoken with your doctor. She'll check on you in the morning. Okay?"

"That'll be fine." He smiled and nodded, as if he'd known my efforts would yield no answers.

He didn't mention the devil, his dead wife, or the fiery path he'd been walking.

I stood, transfixed by this calm old man. Perhaps someday, when I'm an old man wearing a robe with blue piping and cordovan slippers, I'll walk a similar fiery path. Then I may understand what he's tried to tell me. But I was only forty-two, and standing there in my scrubs and stethoscope, I had no insights to ease his pain. I couldn't even tell him why he had a fever.

The overhead speaker crackled. "We need a doctor in room twenty-seven. *Now.*"

"I've got to go."

He raised his right hand in a tremulous benediction.

I forgot the old man as I scrambled through the rest of the shift, grateful to make it to eleven without running across an ectopic pregnancy, or a case of meningitis.

I got home from work after midnight, and tiptoed upstairs. In my sons' room, John had kicked his covers into a tangle around his feet, and Sam was at the end of his bed, without a pillow. I straightened them up, tucked them in, and went to check on Sarah. Her breathing was as quiet as moonlight.

In our room, Sally slept curled on her side. The contours of her hips and shoulders glowed in the streetlight filtering through the curtains. I undressed, and slipped in beside my wife. Lying naked in the pocket of her warmth, I thought about the old man, and the fiery path he'd talked about. I tried to imagine living alone and sleeping by myself, without feeling the mattress shift as Sally moved, without the soothing whispers of her breathing. *What had the old man been trying to tell me, beneath the cool fluorescent lights of the ER?* I'd kept my focus on his fever, even though he'd wanted to talk about the vows he'd carried and the loneliness he'd been left with. Had he just needed to unburden, or was he warning me of a path that could explode into flame, even as I walked it?

Sally and I planned to grow old together. If our marriage succeeded, someday she'd bury me, or I'd bury her. That's how it works. One of us would wake up the next morning and lie motionless in bed, bewildered by the inevitable loneliness that had always seemed impossible.

Sally shifted in her sleep and murmured something I couldn't understand. I eased my head down into my pillow. There was nothing I could do about the old man's loneliness or the warning he'd tried to give me, so I did the only thing I knew to do—I moved closer to Sally's warmth. The subtle, complex scent of her sleeping body calmed me. I slowly breathed in, and out, hoping that sleep would come quickly.

ROTATING SHIFTS

I WAS sitting at the nurses' station, writing a set of discharge instructions, hoping to get out on time. I thought I might even get out a little early.

Barry leaned against the counter of the nurses' station, completing his trip sheet. He was waiting for the charge nurse to tell him where to put his patient—a middle-aged woman sitting on his stretcher, her head propped up as though on a chaise longue. The woman's husband stood close to the gurney, jingling the keys in his pocket.

The cardiac monitor sitting next to her feet showed the smooth green blips of a normal cardiac rhythm. Joanne was busy talking on a telephone. I looked over at Barry and raised my eyebrows.

"Mrs. Stetson's been having chest pain," he said.

The woman looked straight ahead, as if she hadn't heard Barry talking about her. She kept her hands in her lap, her chubby fingers interlaced.

"Are you still having pain?" I asked her.

She looked over at me, and shook her head. "No."

I glanced at the clock—9:57. I was scheduled to leave at 11:00. If Mrs. Stetson was having a heart attack, things could get bumpy, but it would be quick. She sure didn't *look* like someone having a heart attack. And if she wasn't having a true emergency, she could represent a time-consuming problem: she'd want to stay in the hospital and no one would want to admit her. I really didn't want to stay late. "How long did it last?" I asked.

"Fifteen minutes," she said. "Maybe twenty."

"Did you get short of breath?"

"Just a little."

"Any pain in your jaw or arm?" I was looking for associated symptoms.

"Not really."

Joanne kept the phone to her ear, nodding quickly, as if trying to make the person on the other end of the line hurry up. Holding a finger up to Barry, she scanned the board for a place to put Mrs. Stetson. She hung up the phone, turned to Barry, and said, "Room twenty-six."

"Thanks." Barry straightened up and looked at me. "Want this?" He held out a piece of paper.

I'd already talked with her, so I felt obligated. I reached out. The paper was a Discharge Instruction Sheet dated two days previously: She'd just been in the hospital.

Barry pushed Mrs. Stetson toward the cardiac room.

I handed the paper to Carol, the ward clerk. "Could you print off a Discharge Summary from this admission, and put Mrs. Stetson in for a cardiac work-up?"

The Discharge Summary would help move things forward. If her recent admission had been for chest pain, and if they'd done a cardiac cath, there wouldn't be much of a reason to admit her. Once we have pictures of normal coronary arteries, there's not much left to do, as long as you're confident that it isn't one of the other life-threatening causes of chest pain, such as thoracic aortic dissection, or pulmonary embolism. Of course, Mrs. Stetson had arrived with red lights and sirens, so it could be hard to pat her on the shoulder and send her back out. Her husband would look at me reproachfully, shake his head, and say, "*Something's* wrong." He'd nod toward his wife. "She doesn't come running to the hospital with every little pain."

I went into Mrs. Stetson's room. Her husband stood at the head of the bed, scowling. Hopefully it was from worry, not anger.

I introduced myself. "Your chest was hurting for about fifteen or twenty minutes?"

"More like half an hour," the husband said.

I looked over to Mrs. Stetson. "Would you say it was closer to half an hour?"

"Maybe."

I asked about associated symptoms and cardiac risk factors. "You were recently admitted for chest pain?"

"Yes," she said. "They weren't sure what was causing it."

"Did they do a cardiac catheterization?"

"No," she said. "They did a stress test."

Her husband crossed his arms over his chest.

Since they hadn't done a cath a couple of days ago, I knew I could get her admitted without much hassle. They could observe her overnight, and cath her first thing in the morning. "We'll get an EKG, and some labs. Depending on what they show, we can admit you or let you go home with close follow-up with your regular doctor."

"If there's any doubt," her husband said, "I'd rather you keep her."

"Let them decide," Mrs. Stetson said. "They're the doctors."

"Everyone gets to vote," I said. I'll never know, but I've often wondered what would have happened if I'd asked for Mrs. Kelly's vote before I sent her husband home. "Let's get the work-up started, and think in terms of admitting you for observation." I examined her, listening to her heart and lungs carefully. The EKG tech wheeled into the room as I finished the physical exam. I waited as the machine spit out a piece of red graph paper, with the lines of the EKG squiggling across, left to right. I pulled the paper free from the machine, and looked at the tracing. "It's normal," I told Mrs. Stetson and her husband. "But we should still probably watch you overnight."

"Let's do that," her husband said.

I gave Mrs. Stetson an aspirin, and an inch of nitroglycerin to make sure she didn't have any more chest pain, sent off all the labs, dictated an ER note, and started working on getting my other patients admitted, or sent home.

About thirty minutes later, Robert, the nurse, said, "Paul, Mrs. Stetson's having more chest pain. This is her rhythm strip." He handed me the narrow white strip of graph paper with the patient's tracing. The ST segments, the flat parts following the tall spikes, were elevated. "Huh," I said. "Get a twelve-lead EKG." The ST segments of a rhythm strip may or may not mean anything. If the EKG showed ST segment elevation, Mrs. Stetson was having a heart attack. "And start her on a nitro drip. And start another line," I said.

I walked into the room.

Mrs. Stetson's face was pale, and she was sweating. "I'm gonna die," she said.

"Not tonight," I said. "You're going to be fine." I crossed my arms and tried not to fidget while the EKG tech stuck little tabs across the patient's chest, and hooked up her machine.

Robert and Laura were waiting until the EKG was done before starting the second IV line. If the patient moves, or jiggles, the EKG jiggles, too. The EKG tech was waiting for the wavy line to settle down. "Take whatever you can get," I told her. I could see on the screen of her machine the pattern of a myocardial infarction, and didn't want to wait for a perfect EKG. The technician sighed loudly, pushed a button, and the red-lined graph paper slowly advanced from her machine.

She tore it off and handed it to me. *Big MI.* "Ma'am," I said, looking across at Mrs. Stevens, "the EKG shows you're having some blockage in one of the arteries feeding your heart."

She stared at my face.

"And we're going to need to open it up, either with a clot buster medicine, or in the cath lab," I said.

"Is it serious?" her husband asked.

"Yes, it is," I said. "When there's a blockage, it causes a heart attack. If we can get the blockage open, there won't be as much damage. So, we're going to have to work fast, okay?"

They both nodded.

"I need to do a rectal exam," I said, putting on a pair of gloves "to make sure you don't have any bleeding that would make the clot buster more dangerous." She lifted her hips, and I pulled her underwear down just enough to sneak a finger into her rectum. Brown stool, no blood. I daubed a little stool on the card to test for occult blood. "Negative," I called out, so the nurses could record it, too.

I paged the cardiologist, who suggested a thrombolytic, the clot buster, because we could get it in quicker than they could get the cath team in. I told Robert we were going to thrombolyze her, and he called down to the pharmacy to get the drugs.

With the drugs on the way, I went back and explained to Mrs. Stetson the risks and benefits of the clot buster. I showed them the EKG, pointing out the nice, flat ST segments on the initial EKG from when she arrived, and the tall, dome-shaped ST segment of the second EKG. I knew they wouldn't understand the electrophysiology, but they seemed to like seeing the EKG. I didn't tell them that as a resident we'd call the dome-shaped ST segments "tombstone changes," reflecting their shape, and their ultimate effect, if left untreated.

We got the clot-dissolving medication in quickly, and her ST segments began to normalize. Mrs. Stetson's husband was the first to notice, on the monitor on the wall. "Are those places that are supposed to be flat going back down?" he asked, pointing to the monitor.

"Looks like," I said. "Let's check." I ordered a repeat twelve-lead EKG, which showed the ST segments were starting to normalize. *Cool.* Her chest pain was better, too.

"You were right," I said, pointing to the EKG. "They're almost back to where they were."

Mrs. Stetson and her husband looked at the tracing, then to me.

"Were you scared?" Mrs. Stetson asked me.

"Concerned? Yes." I shook my head. "Scared? No." I smiled. "You're in the right place." I nodded toward Robert and Laura, in the room with me. "And you've got good nurses."

Disaster averted, Mrs. Stetson became chatty. "Are you here all night?" she asked me.

"I go home at eleven."

She and her husband looked up at the clock on the wall. It was 11:20. "You're not going to leave before the cardiologist arrives," her husband said, "are you?"

"I'll wait for Dr. Turner," I said. "She'll be here soon."

"Thanks," Mrs. Stetson said. "I appreciate it."

I was glad that the shift had been slow enough to spend some time in the room, show the EKG to the patient and her husband.

Dr. Turner came in, and arranged for the patient's admission to the intensive care unit.

I got out of the hospital about midnight, but felt good about it. Emergencies are fun, when they go well.

When I got home, I opened a Moosehead, and tiptoed into the bedroom. Sally was in the bathroom. "How was your night?" she whispered, as if not wanting to wake herself all the way up.

"Good," I answered, in the same soft voice. "Had a lady come in with chest pain, thought she was bullshitting." I stripped out of my scrubs. "Then she infarcted right there in front of us."

Sally nodded sleepily, and flushed the toilet.

"We got the thrombolytic in, and her ST segments were coming down before she went to the unit."

"Good," she said. She kissed me on the lips, her mouth tasting sleepy, her cotton gown brushing against my naked skin. Then she climbed back into bed.

The next morning, Sally's van was gone: running errands or something. She came home at about eleven.

"You're up," she said, walking into the kitchen.

"Yup." I sipped my coffee.

"Did you tell me about a patient with a heart attack last night?"

We took our coffee to the screened porch, and sat in the white wicker chairs. The air was almost cool enough to make goose bumps on my arms, and the morning sun splayed warmly through the railings between the screens. I told Sally the whole story about the woman with the MI, and how I had enough time to talk with her and her husband. When we'd finished our coffee, Sally said, "I'm still sleepy. Think I'll take a nap."

For the last several months we'd been making love with a giddy, newfound urgency. Was it a quirk of menopause, the result of having all the kids in school, or a deepening trust from so many years of marriage? Neither of us knew, but we'd decided to enjoy it for as long as it lasted.

I went to her and kissed her, barely brushing my lips against hers.

She raised her eyebrows, smiling again. "How about you? Sleepy?"

"Not really." I kissed her again. "But if you'd like some company."

She laughed and pulled me to the bed.

Afterwards, we lay facing each other.

"I'm glad you work rotating shifts," Sally said.

"Huh?" I frowned, and pulled away. Rotating shifts leave me chronically sleep-deprived. I live a jet-lagged life.

"Sometimes it's hard to make love well at night." She touched my cheek. "You know, after getting the kids to bed and everything." She smiled. "I like having some time together in the mornings."

"Me, too." I kissed her.

"I think I'll take that nap I was talking about," Sally said, without opening her eyes.

I slipped out of bed, switched on the white noise machine to the sound of a waterfall—a soothing, subtle roar—and climbed back in bed with my wife.

EPILOGUE

My schedule bounces me through night and day like a pinball. Time blurs into a confusing haze. Often, the ER I walk into is more chaotic than the schedule that put me there. A drunk vomits over the side of his stretcher as another man screeches in pain. Sometimes I feel as though I've stumbled into a painting by Hieronymus Bosch. People come in with trivial complaints: they need a work note, or they took Tylenol Cold & Flu and still have a sniffle, and they tell us to "hurry up." They call the nurses "bitch." I've been called "motherfucker" several times. ("That's "Dr. Motherfucker to you, sir.")

The ER offers steady work; the house isn't paid for; and I'd like to help the kids pay for college. But I could support my family with a less stressful job. I stay because I like the people I work with: they're some of the funniest, hardest working, and most caring people I've ever known. And it's hard to remain compassionate at two o'clock in the morning when your patient is hostile, and you're tired, and you really don't like the guy.

The nurses and docs in the ER don't make a big deal about what they do. Neither do the ward clerks, nursing assistants, or housekeepers. We just do our jobs.

The ER is changing me. When I started out as a nursing assistant, I was emotionally engaged and eager to help. I was afraid I'd never know enough to be useful in an emergency. But I'm proud of the competence I've acquired, and grateful to the people who trained me. And I've come to think that compassion isn't an emotion. It's an action. A discipline.

I'm still trying to decide how emotionally porous I should be. I've joked about wanting a set of scrubs made of Kevlar coated with Teflon: I'd be bulletproof, and nothing would stick—blood, spit, and curses would all slide right off. But I've come to think that a more nuanced response is better: Like the aperture of a camera that opens and closes, I'm learning to vary my emotional permeability. Sometimes, a hard glaze is needed to squeak a patient through a tight spot; other times, I need to open up to acknowledge someone's pain, or fear. I've come to think that this is the only way I can keep doing this work, but it takes practice, and I'm still learning how to do it.

Imagine a floppy three-month-old who will die without intravenous medications and fluids. The most skillful nurses in the department have tried, and failed, to establish an IV. The life-saving intervention is to hold the chubby little leg in your left hand, and with your right hand, force a needle the size of a sixpenny nail down through the skin and muscles and into the bone itself. In the Advanced Pediatric Life Support classes, we practice on chicken legs. You feel a crunchy little "pop" as the needle breaks through the cortex, and into the bone. If the needle wiggles, you're not into the bone—it should feel solid, as if you'd driven it into wood. It's brutal, but it works. I've had to do it to infants a couple of times, and I focused exclusively on the spike and the bone I was driving it down into. No emotion. No hesitation. But when I talked to the mother, her face colored by fear, I needed to soften the edge I'd brought forward to help me resuscitate her child.

The effort of opening and closing the emotional aperture twenty times a day is exhausting, but the other options are not sustainable. If my only response was cynical detachment, I'd lose connection with my family, coworkers, and patients. If I remained fully open to the pain and risk around me, I'd be paralyzed, unable to spike a needle into an infant's leg—or to poke a three-inch needle into an adult's groin, probing to find the deep vein that runs there.

After four years of medical school, three years of training, and thirteen years in practice, I have acquired the technical skills that are necessary to do my job, and am gaining the emotional and spiritual insights that allow me to continue it. I feel as though I'm settling into the life I always hoped I'd have. At work, I weave through night and day, and I know every hour on the clock. I dip into people's lives for brief but important slivers of time. Most shifts, I bring some order to the chaos and some comfort to the pain. I'm learning to call that close enough.

ACKNOWLEDGMENTS

FIRST, and forever, I thank Sally. For marrying me. For bringing her calm, humor, and courage to our marriage. For encouraging me to write. Our agreement was that I could write whatever I wanted, and she could delete whatever she wanted. I also appreciate the encouragement I received from our children, Sarah, John, and Sam. In telling my story, I had to tell parts of theirs. I have written as honestly and as thoughtfully as I could. I hope that my family will be as forgiving of this book's flaws as they've had to be of mine.

My brother, Mark, has encouraged my writing ever since I started. Thank you, Mark. I also want to thank my mother, Betty Austin, and my father, Neal Austin.

I am grateful to my agent, Michelle Tessler, for believing in my writing, and to the folks at W. W. Norton. I couldn't believe my good fortune when Jill Bialosky took on my book. I admire her gifts as a writer of poetry and prose, and she has edited some of my favorite books of all time. I am thrilled that she edited this one. I am grateful that she saw value in my writing and turned my manuscript into such a beautiful book. Paul Whitlatch, her editorial assistant, was skillful and kind as he shepherded the book, and me, through a process I had no experience in. Adrienne M. Davich, another editorial assistant, took over midway through and provided seamless care of the book. Samantha Choy did an excellent job as the book's publicist. Ann Adelman did an incredible job as the book's copy editor: if any errors in punctuation, usage, or spelling slipped past her, it was because she had so many coming at her at the same time. The design team did a wonderful job. I do not think that any writer, anywhere, at any time, could be happier than I am with the way the book turned out.

This book never would have happened without the North Carolina Writers' Network. Knowing a bunch of good stories is one thing. Being able to write them is another. The ER provided the stories, and the NCWN taught me how to write them. The following teachers have helped me, in classrooms, workshops, and by critiquing my work, from the very beginning. I cannot adequately express my gratitude to: Maudy Benz, Abigail Dewitt, Philip Gerard, Judy Goldman, Virginia Holman, Ruth Moose, Peggy Payne, and Saundra Redding.

Another teacher, to whom I will be forever grateful, is Ernie Rancourt. He taught me English in the twelfth grade. He also taught me how to live. I would also like to thank Frank Overton, who helped me grow as a person and as a writer.

I will always be grateful for the Bread Loaf Writers' Conference, and to Michael Collier, the director; Jennifer Grotz, the assistant director; and Noreen Cargill, the administrative manager. They have consistently put together a conference that is unparalleled. The following faculty and fellows have been kind enough to find value in my work, and have been more than generous, as they've helped me grow as a writer: Amy Benson, David Bradley, Peter Chilson, Rachel Cohen, Ted Conover, Rachel DeWoskin, William

Kittredge, Debra Marquart, Sebastian Matthews, Susan Orlean, and Dana Sachs.

My coworkers in the ER—nurses, docs, nursing assistants, ward clerks, housekeepers, respiratory therapists, X-ray techs—have been very supportive over the course of the seven years I've been working on this book. Their interest and support made it easier to keep writing, even when it seemed futile. The following coworkers have given me specific feedback on the manuscript, which was very helpful: Jack Allison, Mary Amato, Kiara Eily, Sam Grossinger, Jodie Johnson, Jon Jones, Ted LaMay, Albert Malvehey, Ron McLear, Mike Minogue, Todd Rogers, Cynthia Shimer, Eugenia Smith, Paul Wiegand, and Hank Wright.

Friends that have read the book and given feedback include: Cathy and Jim Dykes, Sarah Stern, Candy and Mike Webster, Gin Wiegand, and Sue Wilson.

I would also like to thank my patients and their families. Most of them are thoughtful, kind people, who appreciate whatever care my coworkers and I can offer. After reviewing what I've written, I see that I haven't included many of those patients—people who tell me not to worry when I apologize for how long they've had to wait, people who encourage me to take care of the sicker patients first. These people have no way of knowing how much their patience and understanding help during a busy shift. I'll have to start telling them.